# ANKYLOSING SPONDYLITIS

Other titles in the *New Clinical Applications* Series:

**Dermatology** (Series Editor Dr J. Verbov)
   *Dermatological Surgery*
   *Superficial Fungal Infections*
   *Talking Points in Dermatology – I*
   *Treatment in Dermatology*
   *Current Concepts in Contact Dermatitis*
   *Talking Points – II*

**Cardiology** (Series Editor Dr D. Longmore)
   *Cardiology Screening*

**Rheumatology** (Series Editors Dr J. J. Calabro and Dr W. Carson
Dick
   *Ankylosing Spondylitis*
   *Infections and Arthritis*

**Nephrology** (Series Editor Dr G. R. D. Catto)
   *Continuous Ambulatory Peritoneal Dialysis*
   *Management of Renal Hypertension*
   *Chronic Renal Failure*
   *Calculus Disease*

# NEW
# CLINICAL
# APPLICATIONS
# *RHEUMATOLOGY*

# ANKYLOSING SPONDYLITIS

Editors

## JOHN J. CALABRO
MD, FACP

Professor of Medicine and Pediatrics
University of Massachusetts Medical School
Director of Rheumatology
Saint Vincent Hospital
Worcester, Massachusetts, USA

## W. CARSON DICK
MD (Glas.), MBChB, FRCP (Lond.)

Department of Rheumatology
Royal Victoria Infirmary
Newcastle-upon-Tyne
NE1 4LP, UK

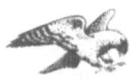 **MTP PRESS LIMITED**
a member of the KLUWER ACADEMIC PUBLISHERS GROUP
LANCASTER / BOSTON / THE HAGUE / DORDRECHT

Published in the UK and Europe by
MTP Press Limited
Falcon House
Lancaster, England

*British Library Cataloguing in Publication Data*

Ankylosing spondylitis.—(New clinical
  applications. Rheumatology).
  1. Ankylosing spondylitis
  I. Calabro, J. J.   II. Dick, W. Carson
  III. Series
  616.7'3     RD771.A5

  ISBN-13: 978-94-010-7950-1     e-ISBN-13: 978-94-009-3231-9
  DOI: 10.1007/978-94-009-3231-9

Published in the USA by
MTP Press
A division of Kluwer Academic Publishers
101 Philip Drive
Norwell, MA 02061, USA

*Library of Congress Cataloging in Publication Data*

Ankylosing spondylitis.

  (New clinical applications. Rheumatology)
  Includes bibliographies and index.
  1. Ankylosing spondylitis.   I. Calabro, John J.
II. Dick, W. Carson (William Carson)   III. Series.
[DNLM: 1. Spondylitis, Ankylosing. WE 725 A6112]
RD771.A5A65   1987     617'.375     87–17297

# CONTENTS

# LIST OF AUTHORS

*J. J. Calabro, MD, FACP*
Professor of Medicine and
Pediatrics,
University of Massachusetts
Medical School,
Director of Rheumatology,
Saint Vincent Hospital,
Worcester,
MA 01604, USA

*A. J. Freemont, MD, MRcP,
MRcPath*
Department of Rheumatology,
University of Manchester
Medical School,
Stopford Building,
Oxford Road,
Manchester M13 9PT, UK

*J. T. Gran, MD*
Lillehammer Rheumatism
Hospital,
2600 Lillehammer, Norway

*G. Husby, MD*
Department of Rheumatology,
University Hospital of Tromsø,
9012 Tromsø,
Norway

*J. Jiminez, MD*
Associate,
Department of Rheumatology,
Hospital General del Centro,
Médico Nacional,
IMSS,
Mexico City,
Mexico

*M. A. Khan, MD, MRCP*
Associate Professor of Medicine,
Case Western Reserve
University,
Cleveland Metropolitan General
Hospital,
3395 Scranton Road,
Cleveland,
Ohio 44109, USA

*G. Mintz, MD, FACP*
Professor and Chairman,
Department of Rheumatology,
Hospital General del Centro,
Medico Nacional,
IMSS, Av. Cuauhtémoc 330,
Mexico City,
Mexico 06725

# SERIES EDITORS' FOREWORD

Ankylosing spondylitis, the third most common form of chronic arthritis, is a systemic rheumatic disorder characterized by inflammation of the axial skeleton (spine and sacroiliac joints), and a host of systemic manifestations. With comprehensive care, the vast majority of patients can lead full, productive lives. However, management can succeed only with patient education and exercise.

Recent communication from my co-editor, Carson Dick, serves to remind me that there are several unresolved issues concerning drug therapy in ankylosing spondylitis. Clearly, in spite of my views, there are others who do not believe that the non-steroidal anti-inflammatory drugs (NSAIDs) alter favorably the course of disease and they must be administered for prolonged periods and in anti-inflammatry quantities to be effective. I would agree with Carson Dick that aspirin and phenylbutazone are way down the list of drug priorities following the marketing of other NSAIDs that are effective and safer.

I am grateful to my contributors to this volume, all recognized authorities on their particular topic. It has been a privilege collaborating with them on this particular volume.

# ABOUT THE EDITOR

**John J. Calabro,** MD, is Professor of Medicine and Pediatrics at the University of Massachusetts Medical School and Director of Rheumatology at Saint Vincent Hospital, both in Worcester, Massachusetts, USA. He is the author of over 260 scientific articles, including several monographs and a book on arthritis for patients.

Dr Calabro serves on the editorial board of several scientific journals. He is certified by the American Board of Internal Medicine, a fellow of the American College of Physicians and the American Rheumatism Association. He is an affiliate of the Royal Society of Medicine, and a member of the Horseshoe Club of England. He also serves as a consultant to the Food and Drug Administration's Orphan Products Development.

# 1
# PATHOLOGY OF ANKYLOSING SPONDYLITIS

*A. J. FREEMONT*

## INTRODUCTION

There has been increasing interest generally in ankylosing spondylitis (AS) over the past 10 to 15 years. Pathological studies, notably the work of Cruickshank[1-3], Ball[4-6] and Bulkley and Roberts[7], have proved central to our present understanding of this disease. They have firstly demonstrated the inflammatory nature of AS; secondly emphasized the balance between inflammatory tissue damage and subsequent repair in the pathogenesis of the disease and thirdly defined the precise distribution of the inflammatory lesions.

In this chapter the main pathological features of AS will be described under three subheadings: the distribution of the disease, articular manifestations of AS and non-articular lesions.

## DISTRIBUTION OF LESIONS

The recurrent non-specific inflammatory lesions of AS appear to be restricted to synovium, articular capsular and ligamentous attachments to bone (entheses) and, less commonly, the anterior uvea and the root of the aorta. One can only speculate on this tissue specificity, which is also displayed, to a lesser extent, in the spondylitic syndrome associated with Reiter's disease, psoriasis and inflammatory bowel disease (secondary AS), although a genetic link has been demonstrated

1

between uveitis, sacro-iliitis and syndesmophytic enthesopathy in that each of these alone is associated with HLA-B27[8,9].

Other lesions are encountered in AS some of which, such as amyloidosis and fracture, are essentially secondary phenomena, whilst others, for instance pulmonary fibrosis and prostatitis, have a more uncertain relationship to the primary disease process.

## ARTICULAR LESIONS

The articular lesions of AS are either directly inflammatory or secondary to inflammation. The inflammatory lesions are of two types, a synovitis and an enthesopathy.

### Synovitis

#### Synovium

Involvement of diarthrodial joints is very common. The synovium in classical AS shows synoviocyte hypertrophy and hyperplasia and contains a predominantly lymphoplasmacytic infiltrate qualitatively indistinguishable in routine preparations from rheumatoid arthritis (RA). In AS the density of the inflammatory cell infiltrate tends to be less than in RA[10]. Nevertheless, in the synovium in AS, the development of vessels specialized for promoting lymphocyte migration from blood is evidence of a high rate of lymphocyte traffic through the synovium[11]. Immunocytochemical studies show that the synthesis of immunoglobulins by intrasynovial plasma cells tends to be predominantly of IgG and IgA types in AS whereas there is a significant contribution by IgM in RA[10] (Figure 1.1).

The synovial appearances and immunoglobulin subtypes are almost identical in secondary AS although it has been reported[12] that the synovitis of Reiter's disease is characterized by prominent polymorphonuclear cell infiltration especially in the early stages. A subintimal polymorph infiltrate has also been described in the synovium in Behçet's syndrome[13].

2

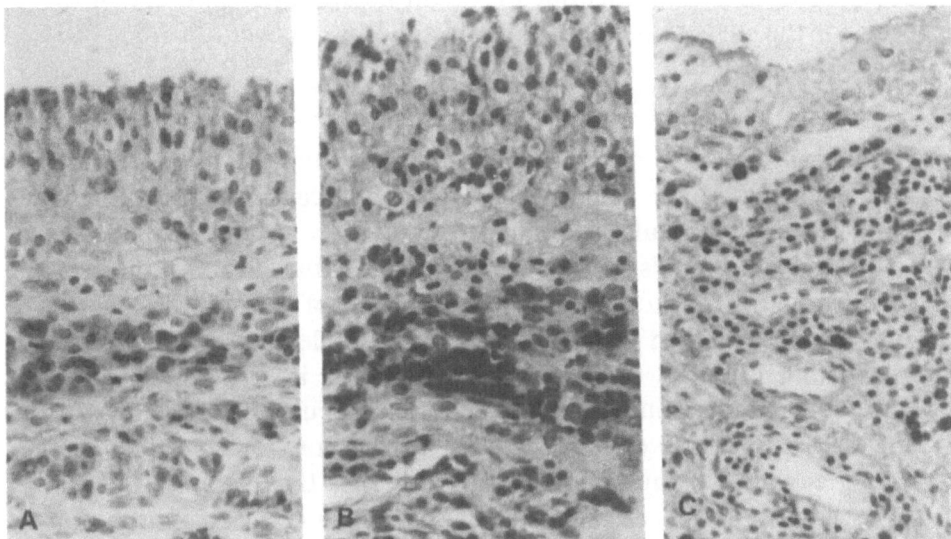

FIGURE 1.1    Synovium in ankylosing spondylitis. A, Stained H & E. B, C immunostaining for IgA and IgM respectively. Note the higher proportion of plasma cells staining for IgA. × 200

## Synovial fluid

On average the synovial fluid polymorphonuclear cell count is lower and the lymphocyte count higher in classical AS than in RA[14]. The peripheral arthropathy in AS is characterized by a high proportion of synovial fluid cytophagocytic mononuclear cells (CPM) – macrophages containing intracytoplasmic degenerate polymorphonuclear cells. Although CPM are not, of themselves, specific for Reiter's disease as was originally suggested[15] only in classical AS and associated disorders such as the arthritis of psoriasis, inflammatory bowel disease and Reiter's syndrome are more than 10% of macrophages cytophagocytic. Mast cells are also a significant feature of the synovial fluid in this group of disorders[16].

Ragocytes, synovial fluid phagocytes containing immunoglobulins and $C_3$[17] in the form of cytoplasmic inclusions, are found in AS but are not as abundant as in RA. The nature of the antigen within the presumptive immune complexes in the ragocyte is unknown but if it could be isolated and identified it might be an important clue in the hunt for the suggested environmental aetiological agent in AS[18].

### Inflammatory enthesopathy

Enthesopathies are lesions of ligamentous and articular–capsular attachments to bone (entheses). In AS the occurrence of enthesopathies in extra-articular sites indicates that these lesions are unrelated to the synovitis. Whilst it has been claimed that the author of the book of Job was the first to describe the symptoms of the enthesopathy of AS[19] we have had to wait in excess of two millennia to the exacting and detailed studies of Ball[4–6] for a reasoned interpretation of the pathology of these and many of the other articular manifestations of the disease. In elective biopsy of focal tender areas over the iliac crest and greater trochanter in patients with AS, Ball showed that the underlying lesion is a non-specific active chronic inflammation concentrated in the enthesis (Figure 1.2). The chondrified and calcified part of the ligament and the bone to which the ligament is attached

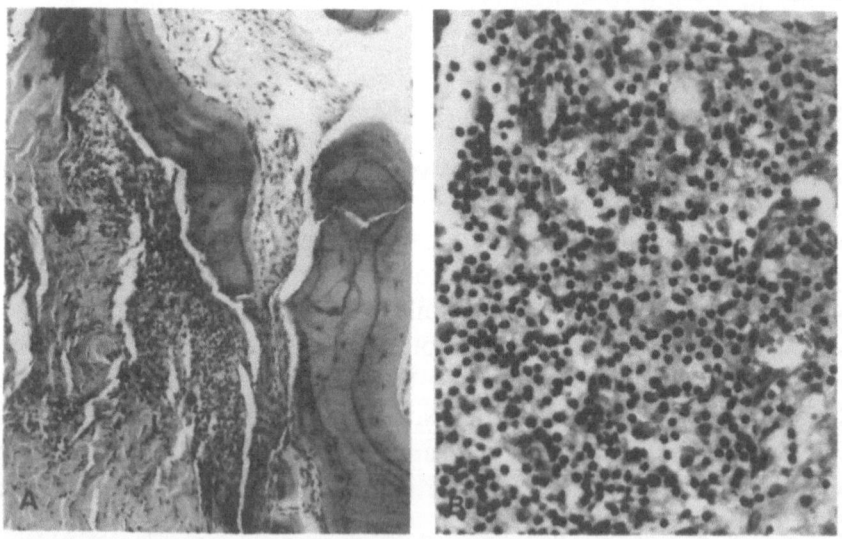

FIGURE 1.2   Erosive enthesopathy. A, Chronic inflammation at the junction of ligament (L) and bone. × 50 B, The chronic inflammatory infiltrate consists of lymphocytes and macrophages together with rare polymorphs. × 200

4

are destroyed and replaced by granulation tissue with a variable infiltrate of lymphocytes, plasma cells and, less frequently, polymorphonuclear cells. Marrow adjacent to the enthesis becomes inflamed and oedematous and loses its haemopoietic cells. The lesions are repaired by direct deposition of reactive (woven) bone which fills in the defect and becomes attached to the eroded end of the ligament to form a new enthesis above the original bone surface. Individual lesions are small but recur, the net result being the gradual formation of a bony spur protruding from the site of the original enthesis into and along the attached ligament (Figure 1.3). During development of the spur the woven bone undergoes remodelling to mechanically stronger lamellar bone.

An enthesopathy may occur in cartilaginous or diarthrodial joints and the formation of bony spurs can lead to ankylosis especially in

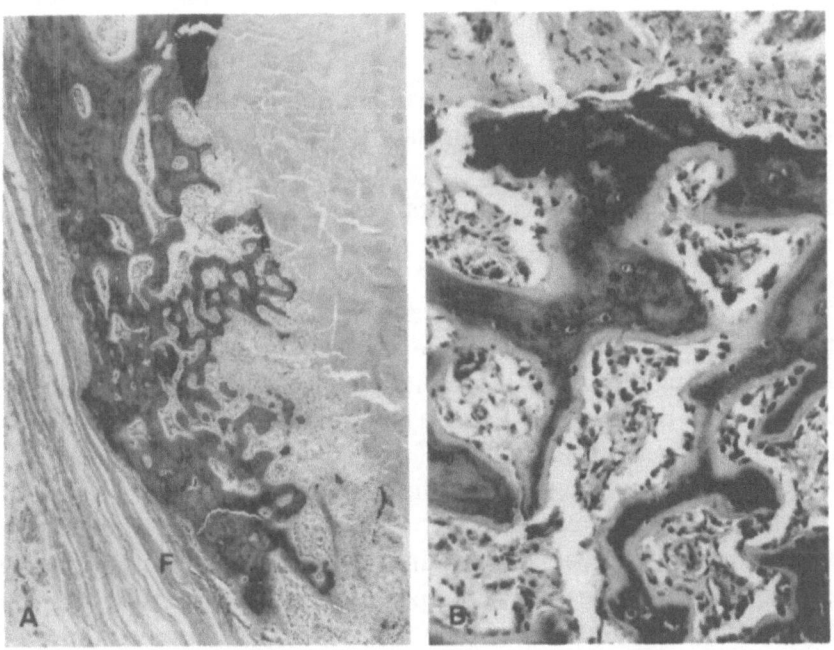

FIGURE 1.3   A, Bony spur within annular fibres (F) of the intervertebral disc. × 15 B, The bone is woven and contains a chronic inflammatory cell infiltrate indicative of a continuing enthesopathy. × 200

joints with relatively low mobility[20], e.g. sacroiliac joints and spinal facet joints.

## Specific features in individual joints

### Cartilaginous joints

*Intervertebral discs.* The enthesopathy occurs at the attachment of the outer fibres of the annulus fibrosus to the anterior and the anterolateral aspect of the vertebral body adjacent to the vertebral rim. Although the erosive lesions are sometimes very small, in many patients they are of a sufficient size to be recognized radiologically[21]. Bony repair leads to the formation of a bony spur known as a syndesmophyte which may ultimately form an ankylosing bony bridge between the rims of adjacent vertebrae. Initially this may be only a few millimetres wide. Syndesmophyte formation is usually followed by a slow but relentless progression to complete ankylosis about the disc. Theoretically this could be due to extension of the enthesopathy but this does not appear to be the case for there is no inflammation during this phase of the disease. It would seem rather that calcification and enchondral ossification of the cartilaginous end-plate, and vascular invasion and ossification within the disc itself are due to some other mechanism (Figure 1.4). Analogy with other lesions strongly suggests this to be the result of the immobilization and changing load transmission across the disc initiated by syndesmophytic ankylosis. Radiological[22] and pathological studies[5] indicate that the disease is multifocal. All segments can be involved with the possible exception of the atlanto-axial joint: indeed in some cervical spines it may be the only joint (including the atlanto-occipital) which is not ankylosed. Ball[6] suggests that this may be because the inherent mobility of this joint either inhibits the development of the enthesopathy or, more likely, its repair and the consequent ossification.

The syndesmophytes described above which extend between vertebral rims are known as 'marginal syndesmophytes'. Rarely syndesmophytes grow beyond the opposite vertebral rim and come to lie alongside, but separate from, the vertebral body. These non-marginal syndesmophytes are usually seen in Reiter's disease and psoriasis, sometimes in the absence of radiologically ascertainable sacro-iliitis[23]. Little is known of the histological appearances of non-marginal syn-

6

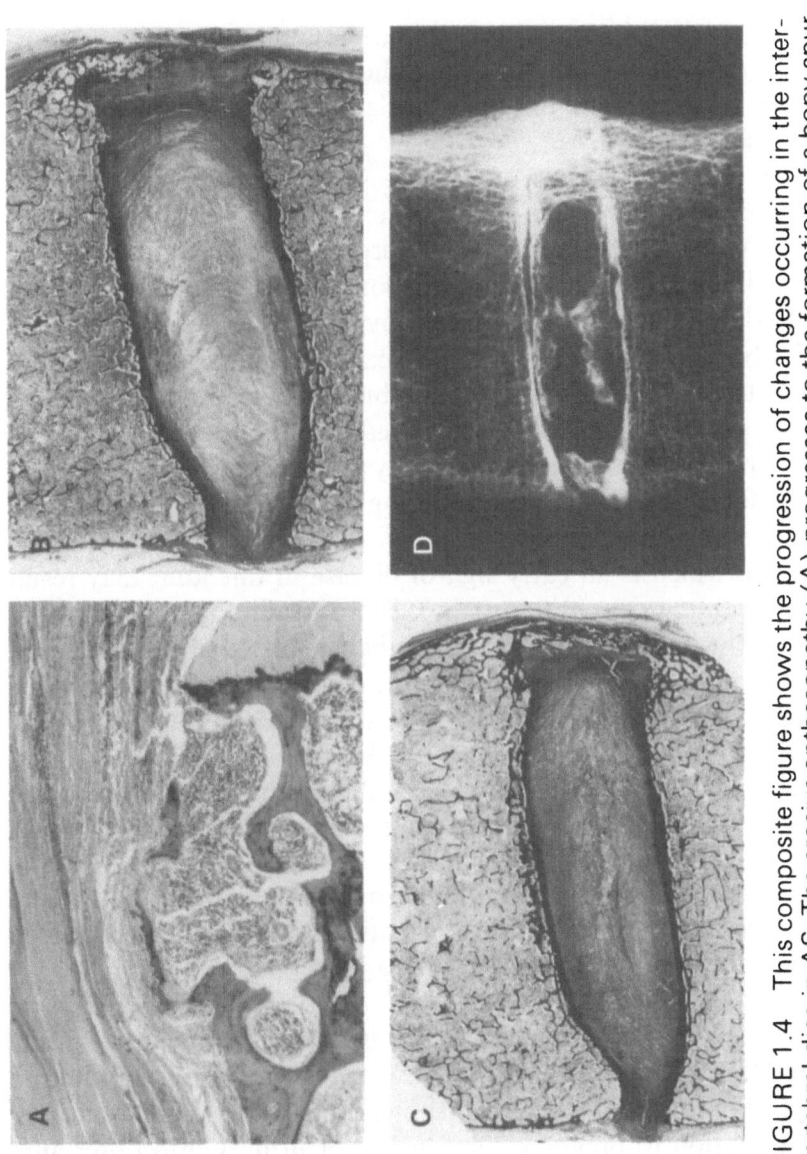

FIGURE 1.4   This composite figure shows the progression of changes occurring in the inter-vertebral disc in AS. The erosive enthesopathy (A) progresses to the formation of a bony spur (B) within the fibres of the annulus. This leads to complete bony ankylosis (C) and, as shown in the slab X-ray (D) subsequent ossification of the disc. A ×12; B & C ×5; D ×3

desmophytes but one case described by Bywaters and Dixon[24] showed them to consist of reactive bone with no apparent associated inflammation.

Atlanto-axial dislocation and spinal fracture may cause neurological complications in AS but otherwise the ankylosing process in the spine is not usually associated with overt neurological disturbances.

*Manubrio-sternal joint.* This joint has certain anatomical and physiological peculiarities which make the interpretation of any pathological changes difficult. First it undergoes spontaneous ankylosis in about 10% of adults[25]; second there are synovial joints between it and the second rib; third a synovium-lined space sometimes forms within the joint itself. Ankylosis of the manubrio-sternal joint occurs in up to half the patients with AS[26]. In some cases a bar of bone resembling a syndesmophyte spans the joint[5]. In many cases, however, the ankylosis takes the form of a synostosis, pathologically indistinguishable from that seen in non-spondylitics.

The pain which is an early sign of disease in this joint may result from an inflammatory enthesopathy[5]. There is radiological evidence of erosion of the joint margins[26,27], and subacute 'osteitis'[1] histologically during this stage of the disease. In Cruickshank's study the periosteal surfaces tended to be involved in the inflammation suggesting the underlying process here might also be an enthesopathy. Other authors[6,27] have described lesions resembling inflammation in synovium-lined clefts and fracture through an old synostosis.

The varied findings in the manubrio-sternal joint may reflect the recognized tendency to synovitis, enthesopathic ankylosis and fracture of ankylosed joints in other sites in patients with AS superimposed upon the morphological vagaries of this joint.

*Symphysis pubis.* The symphysis pubis is another joint in which the interpretation of apparent pathological features can be complicated by 'physiological changes'. In non-spondylitic women erosive changes occur in relation to pregnancy and pelvic or urinary infection[28] and, in normal males radiologically similar changes can follow athletic activity[29]. Having said this Cruickshank[1] described two post-mortem specimens from patients with AS one of which showed a focal erosive osteitis in a narrowed joint with irregular borders and the other narrowing of the joint and bone sclerosis (Figure 1.5).

### Diarthrodial joints

*Apophyseal joints.* In AS a characteristic finding in these joints is synovitis, often accompanied by a minor degree of articular erosion[5,30], and varying amounts of capsular ossification (Figure 1.6). This combination of findings is rare in RA. Both Aufdermaur[31] and Ball[5] conclude that capsular ossification must start at the capsular attachments, and lesions resembling the inflammatory enthesopathy seen elsewhere have also been observed at this site[5]. Capsular ossification can proceed to complete ankylosis. In joints ankylosed by capsular ossification the joint space is usually obliterated and the articular cartilages are in contact forming a so-called synchondrosis. The articular cartilage then undergoes enchondral ossification. Enchondral ossification appears to be a non-specific response of articular cartilage–bone junctions to stress relief. It is seen in diarthrodial joints immobilized by myositis ossificans progressiva[32], in joints relieved of stress experimentally[33] and in the anteromedial part of the femoral head in superolateral osteoarthrosis[34]. The characteristic outcome of the two-stage process of primary capsular ossification and secondary enchon-

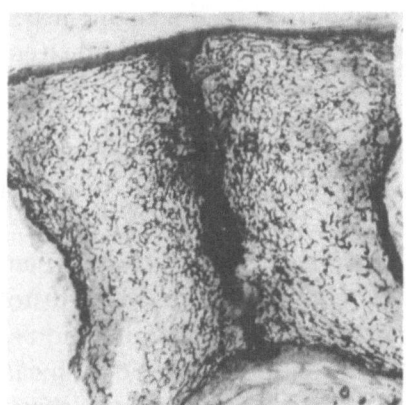

FIGURE 1.5 The symphysis pubis in AS. Bony bridges (B) cross the joint. × 5

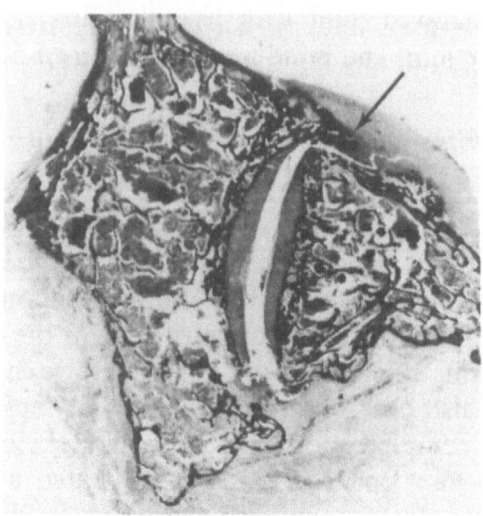

FIGURE 1.6    Apophyseal joint showing capsular ossification (arrowed).
× 12

dral ossification is synostosis with preservation of the joint contours.
A similar outcome is sometimes seen in the hip joint[35] and is characteristic of the sacro-iliac joint (see below).

It is usual for bony ankylosis of apophyseal joints to occur in
conjunction with ankylosis of the corresponding disc. Ankylosis of
costovertebral joints also seems to be associated with ankylosis in
other parts of the segment. Thus if a segment is involved the disease
tends to affect all its component parts whether cartilaginous or synovial.

*Sacro-iliac joints.* There are two histological reports of synovitis in SI
joints of patients with AS[30,36]. Typically, at necropsy the contours of
the sacro-iliac joint are obscured externally by a smooth-surfaced
layer of bone. In the relatively early stages when radiographs show
irregularity of the joint margins, the main histological findings are
peripheral ankylosis due to capsular ossification and enchondral ossification – as in apophyseal joints. The radiological appearances at this
stage are sometimes referred to as 'erosions' because of the irregular
margins of the joint. But histology shows this to be an incorrect
assessment of the pathology. As enchondral ossification occurs it does

10

so at varying rates in different parts of the joint giving rise, in effect, to a series of small bony spurs (Figure 1.7). It is the intervening areas, i.e. the more slowly ossifying segments of cartilage, that are the histological equivalents of the radiological 'erosions'. Subchondral osteitis has not been convincingly demonstrated in either biopsy or necropsy specimens[5,30].

*Temporomandibular joint.* Involvement of the temporomandibular joint in AS has been reviewed by Davidson *et al.*[37]. Biopsy material from one of their patients was reported by Ball as showing an enthesopathy, inflammatory erosive arthritis and secondary degenerative joint disease.

*Other peripheral joints.* In contrast to RA, peripheral arthritis in AS is less erosive and may be associated with radiologically detectable para-articular new bone formation at ligamentous attachments[22,38]. The pathology of this ossifying process has not been reported but as a general rule, it would seem from radiographic studies that in any

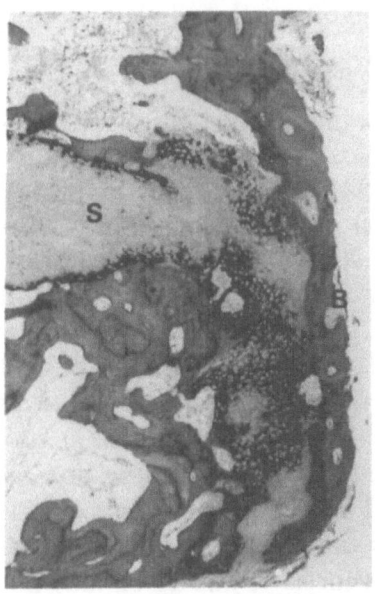

FIGURE 1.7   A bony spur (B) crossing the sacro-iliac joint (S). × 10

synovial joint there is a balance of erosive synovitis and capsular and/or ligamentous ossification and only in joints of low mobility is the ossific process the dominant feature.

## 'Spondylodiscitis'

The disease process in AS typically results in marginal bony ankylosis of intervertebral discs which are otherwise healthy. In some patients, however, there develops a localized or widespread destructive lesion at the disc-bone border. At first these were thought to be infective, but when no organism was identified it was proposed that this might be a severe manifestation of the underlying inflammatory disease process and the lesions were given the title of spondylodiscitis. The most recent studies, however, favour a traumatic aetiology[39].

Clinically, they may be occult but usually the patient presents with localized back pain of a few months duration. Radiologically, localized lesions may be found in either ankylosed or non-ankylosed discs but the most severe lesions are largely restricted to spines with advanced ankylosis. Radiology frequently shows there to be an associated fracture of the neural arch[39], and serial radiographic studies show that destructive lesions involving the whole disc–bone border can follow fracture of the neural arch or an undisplaced complete fracture of an ankylosed segment[40,41]. Similar destructive lesions at the disc–bone border[42] may also be noted following fracture of the neural arch in non-spondylitics indicating that the lesion is a result of trauma rather than AS *per se*. The ankylosed spine is, however, much more susceptible to segmental fracture because of osteoporosis, which is frequently present, the lack of mobility at the discs and variation in the completeness and/or density of the ankylosis at different levels. Should the fracture itself be relatively asymptomatic movement occurring at the fracture site will prevent healing. The patient ultimately presents with what in effect is an ununited fracture or pseudarthrosis and it is this lesion that has often been described as spondylodiscitis.

Severe destructive lesions may occur in non-ankylosed segments of otherwise ankylosed spines in the absence of fracture. It has been proposed by Rivelis and Freiberger[43] in their description of two such cases that the pathogenesis of this lesion may not be so very different from that in the fractured ankylosed segments because here too there

12

would be abnormal stresses and relative hypermobility acting on isolated sections of spine. Destructive lesions in non-ankylosed vertebrae sometimes heal with the formation of massive osteophytes which may obstruct the intervertebral foramina[44].

The histology of various types of destructive lesions is very well described and reviewed by Cawley *et al.*[39]. Briefly, localized lesions in the kyphotic thoracic region were located mainly in the anterior rims which together with the intervening disc was replaced by vascular fibrous tissue (Figure 1.8). The adjacent bone showed oedema, haemorrhage, and variable bone sclerosis but little or no inflammatory cell infiltration. The lesions closely resembled those described by Schmorl and Junghans[42] in elderly non-spondylitic kyphotic individuals. The histology of focal lumbar lesions involving only the vertebral rim has not been reported. However similar, if less severe, lesions have been observed in osteoporotic non-spondylitic spines[45]. Osteoporosis can be present from the earliest stages of AS[46] and it is possible, therefore,

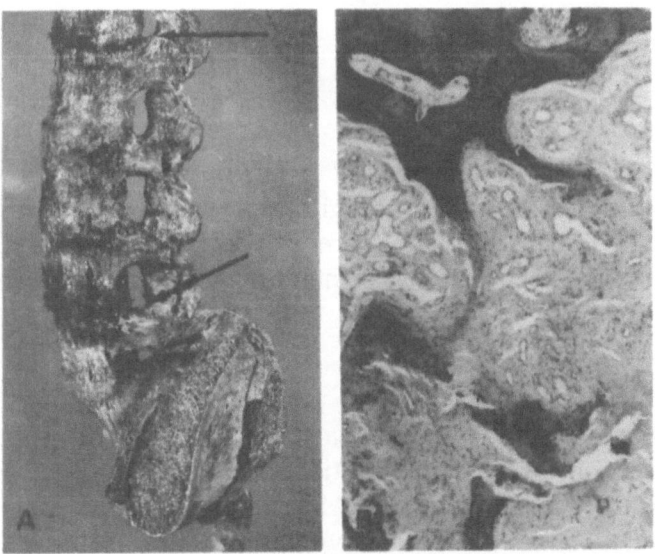

FIGURE 1.8   Traumatic lesions in AS. The macerated spine (A) shows complete bony ankylosis and fractures through the regions of the T12-L1 and L4-5 discs (arrowed). Microscopically (B) there is active granulation tissue and bone destruction. B × 50

that the isolated rim lesions in AS could be a non-specific manifestation of trauma in an osteoporotic spine.

In severe lesions involving the whole disc–bone border the eroded disc–bone interface is replaced mainly by vascular fibrous tissue containing necrotic bone fragments and scanty islands of fibrocartilage. There is no attempt at repair as evidenced by an absence of reactive bone. Active bone remodelling and appositional bone sclerosis are seen in the adjacent vertebral bone, and the marrow spaces in the zone of sclerosis are oedematous and contain small collections of plasma cells and lymphocytes. Since similar if somewhat less conspicuous inflammatory cell infiltration may be seen in ununited fractures in non-spondylitics, the minor inflammatory component, which has also been noted by others[47,48] could be attributed to persistent traumatic tissue damage at the disc–bone border.

Thus, there is a considerable body of evidence, clinical, radiological and pathological that destructive vertebral lesions in AS are essentially due to trauma to a spine which is in various ways rendered unusually susceptible to stress.

## EXTRA-SKELETAL LESIONS

### Ocular

Both classical[8] and secondary[49,50] AS are associated with an acute, unilateral, self-limiting, non-granulomatous anterior uveitis. Although it tends to recur it rarely, if ever, necessitates biopsy or enucleation and its histology has therefore not been fully documented.

### Cardiac

Clinical aortic incompetence and associated disease of the aortic root are observed in up to 10% of patients with classical AS[51,52], and are also encountered in secondary AS[52-54]. Although the pathology is, superficially, similar to that of syphilitic aortitis there are sufficient differences to be found on close examination to render spondylitic aortitis morphologically unique[7].

Macroscopically, the aortic ring and proximal aorta are dilated. The aortic valve cusps are usually fibrotic but the commissures are rarely fused (Figure 1.9). The coronary ostia are patent and may be the site of saccular aneurysms[55].

Microscopically, during periods of active disease, the valve ring and aortic wall contain an inflammatory infiltrate consisting of plasma cells and lymphocytes. It may be associated with fibrous scarring. The inflammatory process and the fibrosis characteristically affect only the proximal few centimetres of the aorta and are maximal in the aortic ring and in the sinuses of Valsalva. This distribution is quite different from that of syphilis and the absence of Aschoff bodies and necrobiotic nodules distinguishes it from rheumatic endocarditis. In the dilated segment of the aorta the functionally important lesion is in the media where there is a focal lymphoplasmacytic infiltrate, destruction of the elastic laminae and reactive fibrosis[51,55]. Replacement of resilient elastic tissue by fibrous tissue almost certainly leads to the aortic

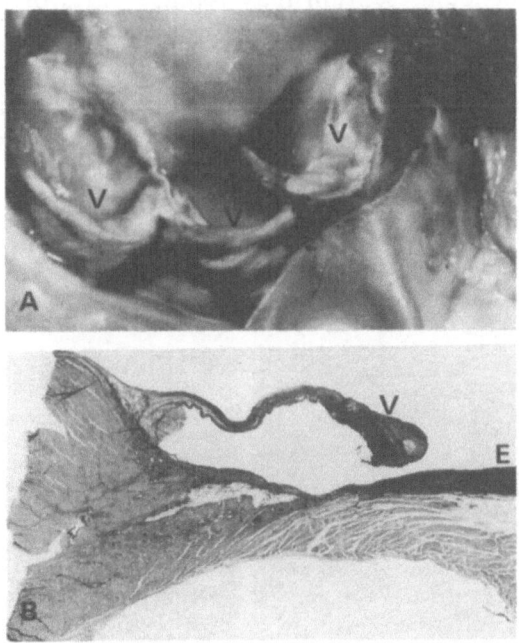

FIGURE 1.9  A, The cusps of the aortic valve (V) are thickened by fibrosis. ×1 B, In this section, stained elastic-van Giesen (EVG), the aortic valve cusp is thickened (V) as is the intima of the aorta (E). ×9

15

dilatation (Figure 1.10). The vasa vasorum do not show a vasculitis but their lumina are narrowed by fibromuscular intimal thickening. The intima and adventitia of the aorta may be thickened by fibrous tissue sometimes containing a chronic inflammatory cell infiltrate. The intimal changes may be widespread in the thoracic aorta but the medial damage is usually localized to the aortic valve and aortic root[55]. Although aortic regurgitation may occur without involvement of the aortic valve[54] it is more usual for the valve cusps to be thickened by vascular fibrous tissue, with or without an inflammatory cell infiltrate. These changes are encountered both at the free margin of the cusp and, unlike syphilis, at its base. Fibrosis may extend below the valve to form a sub-valvular ridge, and into the base of the anterior leaflet of the mitral valve – lesions considered by Bulkley and Roberts[7] to be pathognomonic of AS. Rarely this may result in mitral incompetence[56] but not mitral stenosis.

The myocardium can also contain areas of fibrosis. Fibrous tissue in the interventricular septum may replace parts of the conduction system[57]. This lesion has been observed at necropsy in the absence of aortitis in patients with isolated heart block[52]. It is implicit in clinical reports of spontaneous conversion of heart block to sinus rhythm in patients with AS that there may be a reversible, probably inflamm-

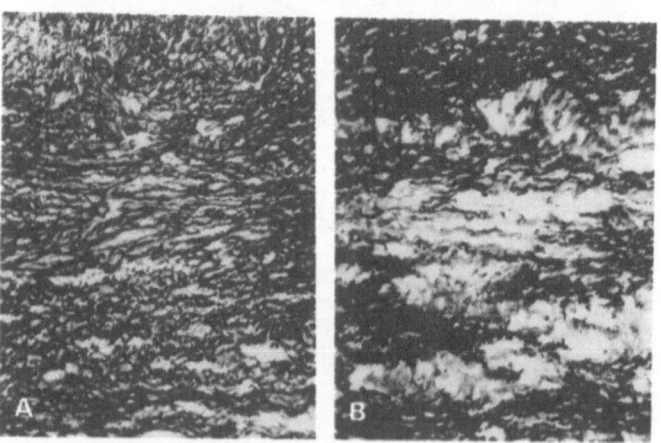

FIGURE 1.10 These are EVG-stained sections of normal aortic media (A) and a similar area (B) from a patient with AS showing destruction of the connective tissue. × 100

atory, early lesion in the interventricular system that may resolve before causing permanent damage[52,54].

## Pulmonary

The prevalence of pulmonary tuberculosis at necropsy (10%), once thought to be high, in patients with AS[58] is no higher than in unselected necropsy populations[3]. However, non-tuberculous upper lobe fibrosis and cavitation is a rare complication of AS. This lung disease first presents many years after the onset of AS[59]. It begins in the apex and in most cases is bilateral. Cavitation develops late in the progression of the disease. The initial lesion is an interstitial pneumonitis in which the alveolar septae are infiltrated by lymphocytes and plasma cells. This progresses to pulmonary and pleural fibrosis, with subsequent bronchiectasis and cyst formation. Secondary fungal infection is a recognized complication.

Although usually relatively trivial, lung involvement of this type is a recognized cause of morbidity and death in patients with AS.

## Renal

Renal function is usually unimpaired in patients with AS[60]. In renal biopsies from non-irradiated patients with normal renal function hyaline arteriolosclerosis and glomerular deposits of immunoglobulin, complement and fibrin have been reported[61,62]. These are probably non-specific findings: Hyaline arteriolosclerosis is a common post-mortem finding even in young adults, and immunoglobulin deposits are known to occur in non-spondylitics in the absence of other evidence of glomerular disease[63].

Renal function impairment does occasionally occur. Rarely a result of IgA nephropathy[64], it is most frequently due to amyloidosis which may progress to renal failure. It is a recognized cause of death in patients with AS. The prevalence of amyloidosis in AS is about 6% as in RA[20]. It is not known why some patients develop this complication but its distribution is typical of the secondary amyloidosis associated with other chronic inflammatory states[65]. There are some intriguing observations which may be of importance when considering the origin of amyloid in AS. First, the prevalence of AS is reportedly

17

increased in Familial Mediterranean Fever – a genetic form of amyloidosis in which arthritis is common[66], and secondly, there is an increased frequency of HLA-B27 in patients with, predominantly seronegative, RA complicated by amyloidosis[67]. These authors suggest that HLA-B27 may be a marker for susceptibility to amyloidosis in patients with seronegative arthritis.

## Prostate

Mason et al.[68] were able to identify significant numbers of neutrophils in fluid obtained by prostatic massage in 45 of 54 patients with AS. They concluded there was an association between AS and prostatitis but could not distinguish cause and effect. This is a provocative observation, particularly in view of the clear association between genito-urinary tract infections, Reiter's disease and secondary AS.

## Nervous system

There are reports of a rare cauda equina syndrome[69,70] which at post-mortem is associated with the formation of periradicular arachnoid-lined diverticulae. In addition some fibrous thickening of the dura and arachnoid have been noted. The pathogenesis of this lesion remains obscure.

Veerapen et al.[71] have recently described a case of AS in which large recurrent osteophytes, probably arising from the apophyseal joints of non-ankylosed segments in the cervical and lumbar spine, caused nerve root compression.

The cerebrospinal fluid protein level is commonly increased in active spinal AS but the cell count is normal[72]. The increase in CSF protein may simply be a reflection of the adjacent process.

## Other organs

Ball[6] has reported a case of AS in which there was a multi-organ vasculitis. This took the form of a necrotizing arteritis in the spleen, pancreas and stomach, resembling that seen in Wegener's granulomatosis. Cruickshank[2], however, in a review series of 439 necropsies on patients with AS identified only two cases with a vasculitis, an almost identical prevalence to control necropsy populations. It seems probable therefore that AS is not associated with disseminated vasculitis.

Involvement of organs other than those specifically mentioned above in the primary disease process of AS is exceptionally rare. Symptoms referable to other organs should alert one to the probability of a co-existent disorder.

## SUMMARY

To date pathological studies have shown that the hallmark of AS is a chronic inflammatory lesion which is episodic, often short lived and highly localized. It accounts for only some of the patients, symptoms and signs. Many of the rest are a consequence of damage to tissues in which non-specific repair processes secondary to inflammation have resulted in loss of specialized elements, leading initially to weakness in, and ultimately structural failure of, connective tissues.

For the future pathological material offers a test system for exploring the aetiology of AS. The unique distribution of the inflammatory lesions may reflect specific epitope expression or antigen homing. Specimens from sites of active inflammation may be ideally suited to the immunohistochemical evaluation of antisera against any putative antigen causally implicated in the disease as, indeed, may the isolated granules of synovial fluid ragocytes.

References

1. Cruickshank, B. (1956). Lesions of cartilaginous joints in ankylosing spondylitis. *J. Pathol. Bacteriol.*, **71**, 73–84
2. Cruickshank, B. (1966). Discussion Arthritis Rounds (5). *Arthritis Rheum.*, **9**, 744–5
3. Cruickshank, B. (1971). Pathology of ankylosing spondylitis. *Clin. Orthop. Rel. Res.*, **74**, 43–58
4. Ball, J. (1968). In Duthie, J. J. R. and Alexander, W. R. M. (eds.) *Rheumatic Diseases*, Pfizer Medical Monographs, No. 3, p. 124. (Edinburgh University Press)
5. Ball, J. (1971). Enthesopathy of rheumatoid and ankylosing spondylitis. *Ann. Rheum. Dis.*, **30**, 213–23
6. Ball, J. (1979). Articular pathology of ankylosing spondylitis. *Clin. Orthop. Rel. Res.*, **143**, 30–37
7. Bulkley, B. H. and Roberts, W. C. (1973). Ankylosing spondylitis and aortic regurgitation. *Circulation*, **48**, 1014–27
8. Brewerton, D. A. (1975). HL-A27 and acute anterior uveitis. *Ann. Rheum. Dis.*, **34** (Suppl. No. 1), 33–5

9. Lambert, J. R. and Wright, V. (1976). Eye inflammation in psoriatic arthritis. *Ann. Rheum. Dis.*, **35**, 354–6

10. Freemont, A. J. and Rutley, C. (1986). The distribution of immunoglobulin heavy chains in diseased synovia. *J. Clin. Pathol.*, **39**, 731–5

11. Freemont, A. J., Jones, C. J. P., Bromley, M. and Andrews, P. (1984). Changes in vascular endothelium related to lymphocyte collections in diseased synovia. *Arthritis Rheum.*, **26**, 1427–33

12. Kulka, J. P. (1962). The lesions of Reiter's syndrome. *Arthritis Rheum.*, **5**, 195–201

13. Vernon-Roberts, B., Barnes, C. G. and Revell, P. A. (1978). Synovial pathology in Behçet's syndrome. *Ann. Rheum. Dis.*, **37**, 139–45

14. Kendall, M. J., Farr, M., Meynell, M. J. and Hawkins, C. F. (1973). Synovial fluid in ankylosing spondylitis. *Ann. Rheum. Dis.*, **32**, 487–92

15. Pekin, T. J., Malinin, T. I., Zvaifler, N. J. (1967). Unusual synovial fluid findings in Reiter's syndrome. *Ann. Intern. Med.*, **66**, 677–84

16. Freemont, A. J. and Denton, J. (1985). The disease distribution of synovial fluid mast cells and cytophagocytic mononuclear cells in inflammatory arthritis. *Ann. Rheum. Dis.*, **44**, 312–15

17. Fehr, K. (1976). In Wagenhauser, F. J. (ed.) *Chronic Forms of Polyarthritis.* pp. 116–5. (Bern: Hans Huber)

18. Geczy, A. F. and Yap, J. (1982). A summary of isolates of Klebsiella Pneumonia which cross-react with HLA-B27-associated cell-surface structure on the lymphocytes of patients with ankylosing spondylitis. *J. Rheumatol.*, **9**, 96–100

19. Jayson, M. I. V. (1983). *NASS Newsletter.* Autumn/Winter

20. Ball, J (1980). In Moll, J. M. H. (ed.) *Ankylosing Spondylitis.* (Edinburgh: Churchill Livinstone)

21. Kinsella, T. D., MacDonald, F. R. and Johnson, L. G. (1966). Ankylosing spondylitis: a late re-evaluation of 92 cases. *Can. Med. Assoc. J.*, **5**, 1–9

22. Dihlmann, W. (1968). *Spondylitis ankylopoetica* – die Bechterewsche Krankheit. (Stuttgart: Thieme)

23. Sundaram, M. and Patton, J. T. (1975). Paravertebral ossification in psoriasis and Reiter's disease. *Br. J. Radiol.*, **48**, 628–33

24. Bywaters, E. G. L. and Dixon, A. StJ. (1965). Paravertebral ossification in psoriatic arthritis. *Ann. Rheum. Dis.*, **24**, 313–30

25. Ashley, G. T. (1954). The morphological and pathological significance of synostosis at the manubrio-sternal joint. *Thorax.*, **9**, 159–66

26. Savill, D. L. (1951). The manubrio-sternal joint in ankylosing spondylitis. *J. Bone Jt Surg. (Br.)*, **33-B**, 56–64

27. Solovay, J. and Gardner, C. (1951). Involvement of the manubrio-sternal joint in Marie-Strumpel disease. *Am. J. Roentgenol. Radiother.*, **65**, 749–59

28. Harris, N. H. (1974). Lesions of the symphysis pubis in women. *Br. Med. J.*, **4**, 209–11

29. Harris, N. H. and Murray, R. O. (1974). Lesions of the symphysis in athletes. *Br. Med. J.*, **4**, 211–14

30. Geiler, G. (1969). Die spondylarthritis ankylopoetica aus pathologisch – anatomischer sicht. *Dtsch. Med. Wochenschr.*, **94**, 1185–8

31. Aufdermaur, M. (1957). The morbid anatomy of ankylosing spondylitis. *Documenta rheumatologia*, Geigy, No. 2

32. Cocchi, U. (1951). Hereditary diseases with bone changes, In Schintz, H. R.,

20

Baensch, W. E., Friede, E. and Uelinger, E. (eds.) *Roentgen Diagnosis*, 5th Edn. (English translation), Vol. 1, p. 644 (London: Heinemann)

33. Thompson, R. C. and Bassett, C. A. (1970). Histological observations on experimentally induced degeneration of articular cartilage. *J. Bone Jt Surg. (Am.)*, **52-A**, 435–43

34. Ball, J., Sharp, J. and Shaw, N. (1978). In Scott, J. T. (ed.) *Textbook of the Rheumatic Diseases*, p. 595. (Edinburgh: Churchill Livingstone)

35. Rutishauser, E. and Jacqueline, F. (1959). Les Coxites rhumatismales. *Documenta Rheumatologica*, Geigy, No. 16

36. Dihlmann, W., Lindenfelser, R. and Selberg, W. (1977). Sakroiliakale histomorphologie der ankylosierenden spondylitis als Beitrag zur therapie. *Dtsch. Med. Wochenschr.*, **102**, 129–32

37. Davidson, C., Wajtulewski, J. A., Bacon, P. A. and Winstock, D. (1975). Temperomandibular joint disease in ankylosing spondylitis. *Ann. Rheum. Dis.*, **34**, 87–91

38. Resnick, D. (1974). Patterns of peripheral joint disease in ankylosing spondylitis. *Radiology*, **110**, 523–32

39. Cawley, M. I. D., Chalmers, T. M., Kellgren, J. H. and Ball, J. (1972). Destructive lesions of vertebral bodies in ankylosing spondylitis. *Ann. Rheum. Dis.*, **31**, 345–58

40. Kanefield, D. G., Mullins, B. P., Freehafer, A. A., Furey, J. G., Horenstein, S. and Chamberlin, W. B. (1969). Destructive lesions of the spine in rheumatoid ankylosing spondylitis. *J. Bone Jt Surg. (Am.)*, **51-A**, 1369–75

41. Yau, A. C. M. C. and Chan, R. N. W. (1974). Stress fractures of the fused dorsolumbar spine in ankylosing spondylitis. *J. Bone Jt Surg. (Br.)*, **56-B**, 681–7.

42. Schmorl, G. and Junghans, H. (1957). The human spine in health and disease, 4th Edn. (New York: Grune and Stratton)

43. Rivelis, M. and Freiberger, R. H. (1969). Vertebral destruction at unfused segments in late ankylosing spondylitis. *Radiology*, **93**, 251–6

44. Dunn, N., Preston, B. and Jones, K. L. (1985). Unexplained acute backache in longstanding ankylosing spondylitis. *Br. Med. J.*, **291**, 1632–5

45. Hilton, R. C., Ball, J. and Benn, R. T. (1976). Vertebral end-plate lesions (Schmorl's nodes) in the dorsolumbar spine. *Ann. Rheum. Dis.*, **35**, 127–31

46. Hanson, C. A., Shagrin, J. W. and Duncan, H. (1971). Vertebral osteoporosis in ankylosing spondylitis. *Clin. Orthop. Rel. Res.*, **74**, 59–64

47. Coste, F., Delbarre, F., Cayla, J., Massias, P. and Beaslay, E. (1963). Spondylites destructives dans la spondylarthrite ankylosante. *Presse Medical*, **71**, 1013

48. Sutherland, R. I. L. and Matheson, D. (1975). Inflammatory involvement of vertebrae in ankylosing spondylitis. *J. Rheumatol.*, **2**, 296–302

49. Wright, V. and Moll, J. M. H. (1976). In Sero-negative polyarthritis. (Oxford: North-Holland)

50. Lambert, J. R., Wright, V., Rajah, S. M. and Moll, J. M. H. (1976). Histocompatibility antigens in psoriatic arthritis. *Ann. Rheum. Dis.*, **35**, 526–30

51. Graham, D. C. and Smythe, H. A. (1958). The carditis and aortitis of ankylosing spondylitis. *Bull. Rheum. Dis.*, **9**, 171–4

52. Kinsella, T. D., Johnson, L. G. and Sutherland, R. I. (1974). Cardiovascular manifestations of amylosing spondylitis. *Can. Med. Assoc. J.*, **111**, 1309–11

53. Zvaifler, N. J. and Weintraub, A. M. (1963). Aortitis and aortic insufficiency in the chronic rheumatic disorders – a reappraisal. *Arthritis Rheum.*, **6**, 241–5

54. Paulus, H. E., Pearson, C. M. and Pitts, W. (1972). Aortic insufficiency in five patients with Reiter's syndrome. *Am. J. Med.*, **53**, 464–80
55. Clark, W. S., Kulka, P. and Bauer, W. (1957). Rheumatoid aortitis with aortic regurgitation. An unusual manifestation of rheumatoid arthritis (including spondylitis). *Am. J. Med.*, **22**, 580–92
56. Roberts, W. C., Hollingsworth, J. F., Bulkley, B. H., Jaffe, R. B., Epstein, S. E. and Stinson, E. B. (1974). Combined mitral and aortic regurgitation in ankylosing spondylitis. *Am. J. Med.*, **56**, 237–43
57. Sobin, L. H. and Hagstrom, J. W. C. (1962). Lesions of cardiac conduction tissue in rheumatoid aortitis. *J. Am. Med. Assoc.*, **180**, 1–5
58. Brown, W. M. C. and Doll, R. (1965). Mortality from cancer and other causes after radiotherapy for ankylosing spondylitis. *Br. Med. J.*, **ii**, 1327
59. Vale, J. A., Pickering, J. G. and Scott, G. W. (1974). Ankylosing spondylitis and upper lobe fibrosis and cavitation. *Guy's Hosp. Rep.*, **123**, 97–119
60. Calin, A. (1975). Renal function in ankylosing spondylitis. *Scand. J. Rheumatol.*, **4**, 241–2
61. Pasternack, A., Tallquist, G. and Martio, J. (1970). Renal vascular changes in ankylosing spondylitis. *Acta Medica Scand.*, **187**, 519–23
62. Linder, E. and Pasternack, A. (1970). Immunofluorescence studies on kidney biopsies in ankylosing spondylitis. *Acta Pathologica et Microbiologica Scand.*, **78B**, 517–25
63. McCluskey, R. T. and Hall, C. L. (1978). Immune complex mediated disease. *Human Pathol.*, **9**, 71–82
64. Jennette, J. C., Fergusson, A. L. and Moore, M. A. (1982). IgA nephropathy associated with seronegative spondylarthropathies. *Arthritis Rheum.*, **25**, 144–53
65. Hobbs, J. R. (1978). Genetic disease and amyloid. *J. Clin. Pathol.*, **31** (Suppl. 12) (Royal College of Pathologists), 128–31
66. Dilsen, N. A. (1973). Ankylosing spondylitis in familial mediterranean fever. *Proceedings of XIII International Congress of Rheumatology*, Kyoto. Abstract No. 364, Excerpta Medica Congress, Series No. 299
67. Pasternack, A. and Tiilikainen, A. (1977). Cited by Russell, A. S. and Barraclough, D. R. E. In Brewerton, D. A. (ed.) *Clinics in Rheumatology*, Vol. 3, No. 2. (London: Saunders), **12**, 365–75
68. Mason, R. M., Murray, R. S. and Oates, J. K. (1958). Prostatitis and ankylosing spondylitis. *Br. Med. J.*, **i**, 748–52
69. Matthews, W. B. (1968). The neurological complications of ankylosing spondylitis. *J. Neurol. Sci.*, **6**, 561–73
70. Russell, M. L., Gordon, D. A., Ogryzlo, M. A. and McPhedran, R. S. (1973). Cauda equina lesio associated with rheumatoid spondylitis. *Ann. Intern. Med.*, **78**, 551–7
71. Veerapen, K., Dieppe, P. A., Veerapen, R. and Griffith, H. B. (1986). The 'last joint' syndrome in ankylosing spondylitis. *Br. Med. J.*, **293**, 368
72. Boland, E. W., Headley, N. E. and Hench, D. S. (1948). The cerebrospinal fluid in rheumatoid spondylitis. *Ann. Rheum. Dis.*, **7**, 195–9

# 2

# HLA AND ANKYLOSING SPONDYLITIS

*M. A. KHAN*

## INTRODUCTION

Study of products of genes present on a region on chromosome 6 known as the Major Histocompatibility Complex (MHC) is providing new insight into many chronic diseases of undetermined aetiology, including rheumatic diseases such as ankylosing spondylitis[1,2] and rheumatoid arthritis[3,4]. The human MHC is called HLA, and it contains a tightly linked cluster of genes that encode for cell surface glycoprotein molecules expressed on the cell membrane of virtually all cells[5-7]. These molecules are involved in cell-to-cell interaction and have been subdivided into two distinct groups called class I and class II molecules[6-8]. The class I molecules are encoded by the HLA-A, -B, and -C loci of the MHC. These molecules display an exceptional degree of genetic polymorphism and are composed of an MHC-encoded heavy – or $\alpha$ – chain that is non-covalently bound to $\beta_2$-microglobulin, a smaller and invariant polypeptide chain encoded by a gene located on another chromosome[5-8]. The class II molecules consist of two glycoprotein chains as well, the larger of the two chains is called $\alpha$ chain and the smaller one is called $\beta$ chain. These two chains are closer in size than those of the class I molecules. Moreover, both $\alpha$ and $\beta$ chains are encoded by genes located in the HLA-D region[7,8].

23

Class I HLA molecules serve as recognition structures for cytotoxic T lymphocytes (CTL). They act as restricting elements for recognition of viral antigens expressed on the surface of virus-infected cells for their lysis by autologous anti-viral CTL[6–8].

One of the landmark advances in medicine during the past fourteen years has been the discovery of the remarkable association of ankylosing spondylitis and related spondyloarthropathies with a class I HLA molecule called HLA-B27[1,2]. This association was first observed in studies in Caucasians where more than 90% of spondylitis patients and about 8% of normal controls were found to possess B27[1,2]; this association was later confirmed in studies of patients belonging to various other racial groups as well[9].

## B27 AND DISEASE ASSOCIATION IN VARIOUS RACIAL GROUPS

The B27 gene is mostly found in Caucasoid and Mongoloid racial groups, and is virtually absent in the racially unmixed populations indigenous to the southern hemisphere, e.g. South American Indians and Australian Aborigines[9,10]. The significant association between B27 and ankylosing spondylitis holds true in all racial groups thus far studied and, in general, there is a direct correlation[9–11] between the geographic distributions of the disease and B27. Table 2.1 summarizes the frequencies of B27 in patients with ankylosing spondylitis and in normal controls among different racial groups. The highest known prevalence of B27 in any human racial group is in Haida Indians, who live mostly in the coastal areas of the Canadian province of British Columbia. They have a 50% prevalence of B27 in the general population, and in one survey 10% of adult males were found to have roentgenographic evidence of sacroiliitis[12–16]. The sacroiliitis prevalence among B27-positive Haida men has been estimated to be 20%, and all known spondylitic male and female patients in one study were found to possess B27[15]. There is no evidence that *Yersinia* or *Shigella* infections might be aetiologically related to such high prevalence of sacroiliitis and spondylitis[17], and Reiters's syndrome is absent or extremely rare. Bella Coola Indians, who also live in the coastal areas of British Columbia, have a 25% frequency of B27 in the general population and a 2% prevalence of sacroiliitis[9,15].

TABLE 2.1 HLA-B27 frequency in Caucasian, Mongoloid and Negroid populations

| Populations | Ankylosing spondylitis | | Normal controls | |
|---|---|---|---|---|
| | No. of patients | B27 (%) | No. of controls | B27 (%) |
| Caucasoid | | | | |
| Euro-Caucasoids ('whites') | 2022 | 79–100 | 16 162 | 4–13 |
| Indians and Pakistanis | 130 | 83–100 | 456 | 2–8 |
| Iranians | 25 | 92 | 400 | 3 |
| Arabs | 32 | 81 | 355 | 3 |
| Jews | 31 | 81 | 456 | 3 |
| Mongoloid | | | | |
| Chinese | | | | |
| Mainland China | 196 | 69–91 | 726 | 2–7 |
| Hong Kong | 77 | 99 | 102 | 4 |
| Taiwan | 75 | 95 | 297 | 9 |
| Singapore | 29 | 97 | 238 | 7 |
| Japanese | 72 | 82 | 208 | <1 |
| Filipino | 17 | 94 | 529 | 5–8 |
| Thai | 71 | 86 | 138 | 5 |
| North American Indians | | | | |
| Haida | 17 | 100 | 222 | 50 |
| Navajo | 5 | 80 | 100 | 36 |
| Bella Colla | 3 | 100 | 129 | 25 |
| Pima | 14 | 100 | 400 | 18 |
| Zuni | | | 158 | 13 |
| Hopi | | | 100 | 9 |
| Mestizo* | 239 | 69–81 | 1404 | 3–7 |
| South American Indians† | | | 440 | 0 |
| Negroid | | | | |
| African blacks‡ | | | 259 | 0 |
| South African blacks | 9 | 22 | 798 | 1 |
| American blacks | 67 | 57 | 1330 | 2–4 |

* They are basically Mongoloid (Asiatic origin) like the rest of the Amerindians, living in Latin American countries, but have had continous admixture of Caucasian (primarily Spaniard) and to a small extent Negroid genes since the sixteenth century.
† Of unmixed ancestry.
‡ From Congo and Zambia, of unmixed ancestry
Adapted from Khan[29] and Khan[9] with kind permission of the publishers· Grune and Stratton, Orlando, Florida, and Raven Press, New York, respectively.

Navajo Indians, who live in northeastern Arizona and are ancestrally related to the Haidas, show 36% prevalence of B27, and a relatively high incidence of Reiter's syndrome (133 cases per 100 000 population per year), and a high prevalence of radiographic sacroiliitis (11%); these figures are much higher than in the Caucasian population[18,19]. It is of much clinical interest that the Hopi Indians, who are the neighbours of the Navajos but are of different ancestral origin, do not show a high frequency of Reiter's syndrome, even though shigellosis is endemic among both of these tribes[18-20]. The frequency of B27 is about 9% in the Hopi general population. Epidemiological and immunogenetic studies of these and other isolated native populations in different parts of the world can lead to clearer understanding of the role of HLA antigens in the pathogenesis of ankylosing spondylitis and elucidation of variations in genetic and non-genetic (environmental) predisposing factors.

The B27 gene is virtually absent in African Negroids of unmixed ancestry, and ankylosing spondylitis is believed to be extremely rare in that group, although accurate prevalence figures are not yet available[9-11,21-27]. At a large hospital in South Africa only eight black patients with ankylosing spondylitis were seen over a period of four years; and it was estimated that in a comparable white population, one would anticipate finding 2000 affected persons[21]. Moreover, these black patients were relatively older at disease onset, none had iritis or a positive family history, and most had severe disease. B27 was found in only one of these eight patients[21]; this HLA antigen is very rare (less than 1%) in the general black population of South Africa[21-23,25]. Population studies in the adjacent countries of Zaire and Zambia have shown absence of B27 in 259 individuals studied[25].

Between 2 and 4% of American blacks in the general population possess B27 as a result of racial admixture during the past few centuries[9,10,25,28,29]. Even before the discovery of the association of ankylosing spondylitis with B27, Baum and Ziff[30] had provided indirect evidence to indicate that the prevalence of ankylosing spondylitis in American blacks is almost 25% that in whites. At our hospital, which provides health care for a population with a 3:2 ratio between whites and blacks, white patients with spondylitis outnumber blacks by a ratio of 5:1, further supporting the suggestion by Baum and Ziff that

26

the disease is relatively less prevalent in American blacks. Thus, the prevalence of ankylosing spondylitis depends upon the racial background of the population and follows, to a large extent, the distribution frequency of B27 in the general population[9–11,16,26].

Most of the original data on the prevalence of ankylosing spondylitis, based on detection of radiographic sacroiliitis with or without clinical evidence of the disease, supported a prevalence of 1.5–2 per thousand in the Caucasian populations[31]. Since the discovery in 1973 of the association between B27 and ankylosing spondylitis, some initial reports suggested that 20–25% of the B27-positive individuals develop the disease[32]. This would imply that 1–2% of the adult Caucasian population in the United States suffer from ankylosing spondylitis. More recent data, however, suggest that the disease prevalence is closer to that observed in the 'pre-HLA' era, and it appears that 1–10% (probably closer to 2%) of the B27-positive adults in the general population are likely to suffer from ankylosing spondylitis, as currently defined[10,31,33–35]. The disease is more common among B27-positive first-degree relatives of spondylitis patients, since 20–30% of them are likely to suffer from it[36].

The disease is more commonly observed in males, and the male to female ratio is 3:1 rather than 10:1 as was frequently cited in the past[35–37]. The strength of the disease association with B27 does not differ between male and female patients with spondylitis[26,38].

## COMPARISON OF B27(+) AND B27(−) ANKYLOSING SPONDYLITIS

Table 2.2 summarizes the comparison of the B27-positive and the B27-negative patients with ankylosing spondylitis. We had observed that acute anterior uveitis is significantly more common in B27-positive patients than B27-negative patients[39] and this has been subsequently confirmed by others[40–42]. The skeletal manifestations of the disease are essentially the same in the two groups, but familial aggregation of the disease is very rare among B27-negative patients[11,27–39,43–46]. It is extremely unusual to observe families with two or more first-degree relatives affected with B27-negative primary ankylosing spondylitis in the absence of psoriasis or inflammatory bowel disease in the family[43,47,48]. Moreover, the mean age of onset appears to be a little

27

TABLE 2.2 Comparison of clinical features of B27-positive and B27-negative patients with primary ankylosing spondylitis

|  | B27( + ) | B27( − ) |
|---|---|---|
|  | All races | Increased in non-Caucasians |
| HLA antigens | B27 | Increased B7 in blacks<br>Increased Bw16(B238) in whites<br>(? IBD* or psoriasis genes) |
| Age of onset | 15–40 y | 18–50 y |
| Familial aggregation | + + | − − (in the absence of IBD* or<br>psoriasis in the family) |
| Acute anterior uveitis | + + | + |
| Skeletal manifestations | + + | + + |

* IBD = chronic inflammatory bowel disease.
Adapted from Khan[37] with the kind permission of Grune and Stratton, Orlando, Florida

later in B27-negative patients than in those carrying the antigen[11,21,39,44]. Presence of the observed differences summarized in Table 2.2 suggests clinical and genetic heterogeneity of ankylosing spondylitis[44].

## B7-CREG antigens

Studies of B27-negative spondyloarthropathy patients of various racial groups in different parts of the world may help provide important clues to the disease pathogenesis. For example, among our B27-negative black patients with primary ankylosing spondylitis, we have observed a subgroup of patients whose disease seems to be associated with B7; these B7-positive patients lack familial aggregation of the disease and they are also relatively older at onset of their disease[46]. Arnett et al.[49,50] in Baltimore have observed that 62% of their white B27-negative patients with Reiter's syndrome, sacroiliitis or spondylitis possess B7, Bw22, or B40; all these antigens, like B27, belong to a Cross-REacting Group (CREG) of antigens called B7-CREG[51]. Therefore they suggested that among B27-negative patients with spondyloarthritis, there is an association with B7-CREG antigens[49,50]. We in Cleveland, as well as some investigators in Europe, have not observed such an association in our B27-negative Caucasian patients with ankylosing spondylitis, Reiter's syndrome, or secondary spondylitis[52]. However, as discussed earlier, we have observed, among our B27-negative American blacks, a subset of B7-positive patients with primary ankylosing spondylitis[46]. We did not have enough B27-negative black patients with Reiter's syndrome to demonstrate any significant association with B7-CREG, although 4 of 11 patients (36%) possessed B7 (2 of these 4 B7-positive patients also had Bw22) as compared to 24% of controls[53]. If we analyse all our B27-negative black patients with various spondyloarthropathies, B7 is present in 15 of 32 patients (47%) and 14 of 59 (24%) B27-negative controls.

## B27-homozygosity

A slight excess of B27 homozygosity has been observed among patients with ankylosing spondylitis as compared to controls by some investigators and not by others[54-59]. Family studies had not been performed to confirm the presence of homozygosity in most of the patients in these studies. In a more recent study[60] of 100 B27-positive patients with ankylosing spondylitis, six patients were found to be apparently homozygous as compared to 2.3% expected. Family studies were performed in 58 of the 100 patients; 10 families showed two separately distinguishable B27 haplotypes and no difference was observed between the prevalence of AS in B27 homozygous and heterozygous family members. Clinical features of the disease show no significant differences between B27 heterozygotes and apparent homozygotes except for a higher frequency among the latter group with regard to peripheral joint involvement (including hips and shoulders)[54], and acute anterior uveitis[56,57,60].

## HLA-A alleles

A slightly increased frequency of HLA-A2 has been observed among spondylitis patients as compared to controls; when results of all these studies are pooled together, a significant increase of HLA-A2 can be demonstrated (relative risk = 1.55)[10,26]. This weak association between A2 and ankylosing spondylitis may be the result of some degree of linkage disequilibrium between A2 and B27. Excess of HLA-A2 has been observed among B27-positive ankylosing spondylitis patients with associated acute anterior uveitis, as compared to the B27-positive spondylitis without associated uveitis[61], but it needs confirmation by study of a larger number of patients.

## HLA-C alleles

Studies by various authors, as summarized by Tiwari and Terasake[10], show an association between ankylosing spondylitis and Cw1 and Cw2 antigens, but it results from a known linkage disequilibrium between B27 and these two C-locus alleles.

## HLA-D/DR alleles

Studies of HLA-D alleles by mixed lymphocyte culture have failed to show any association with ankylosing spondylitis[62]. We studied 7 HLA-DR specificities (DR1 to DR7) in 36 spondylitis patients (28 Caucasians, 8 American blacks) and 76 controls (64 Caucasians and 12 blacks), and observed no significant differences[63,64]. This was confirmed in a similar study of 50 French patients with spondylitis[65].

## MECHANISM OF GENETIC PREDISPOSITION

Since the discovery of the remarkable association between ankylosing spondylitis and HLA-B27 14 years ago, progress in our understanding of the aetiopathogenesis of this disease has been relatively disappointing[66]. Any hypothesis explaining the strong association between B27 and ankylosing spondylitis (which is irrespective of haplotype and race) must accommodate the following findings: not all individuals with B27 develop spondylitis; the presence of B27, even in the homozygous form, is not sufficient to cause the disease; and although the association is stronger in Caucasians than in many other racial groups, a small percentage of Caucasian spondylitis patients lack B27[11,45,47,66,67].

The two major concepts advanced to explain the association between B27 and ankylosing spondylitis are: (a) B27 itself is unimportant, but its coding allele is in strong linkage disequilibrium with another distinct 'illness susceptibility' gene; (b) the B27 antigen itself plays a functional role in disease pathogenesis; this effect might be due to its acting as a receptor for a virus or other environmental agent or by its antigenic resemblance to the environmental factor(s), thereby allowing those factor(s) to persist or trigger an abnormal immune response that results in disease[66]. Neither hypothesis excludes the role of other genes, unlinked to chromosome 6, in the pathogenesis of the disease.

It still remains unresolved whether the major pathogenetic factor is the B27 itself or a closely linked gene, but there is growing evidence, summarized below, that strongly suggests that the B27 gene or its product directly plays a major role in disease susceptibility factor, perhaps in conjunction with additional genetic and environmental (non-genetic) triggering factors[44,45,47,66].

The strong association between ankylosing spondylitis and B27 (and not with other genes of the HLA complex), irrespective of haplotype and ethnic, racial and geographic background, the apparent dominant mode of inheritance, and the finding that B27 cross-reacts with epitopes found on certain bacteria implicated as possible disease-triggering factors, strongly suggest that B27 plays a functional role in disease pathogenesis, either in a direct manner or in conjunction with additional genetic and environmental factors[9,47,66,68,69]. If the major spondylitis gene is not the B27 gene itself but an allele at a closely linked locus, recombinational events between B27 and the linked gene occurring over thousands of years should have weakened the association in at least some of the racial groups (unless one postulates that there is an extraordinarily tight linkage or presence of some genetic mechanism that has been suppressing recombinational events, and that there is a remarkable uniformity in the degree of linkage disequilibrium of the hypothesized linked gene with B27 in various ethnic and racial groups)[47,66].

In families with multiple cases of ankylosing spondylitis, one observes that the disease almost invariably segregates with B27 unless there are some family members with psoriasis or chronic inflammatory bowel disease[44,45,47,48]. No family has yet been observed in which there was a B27-positive and a B27-negative relative affected with *primary* ankylosing spondylitis (unassociated with Reiter's syndrome, psoriasis, or inflammatory bowel disease), along with a clearly *documented* evidence of a genetic recombination close to the B locus in the family. Absence of recombination has been consistently observed in a few families with a B27-positive and a B27-negative affected relative

31

studied so far, thus providing circumstantial evidence against the hypothesis that the putative spondylitis gene is at a locus separate from the B locus.

There is evidence to suggest that the presumed disease susceptibility genes for psoriasis, ulcerative colitis and Crohn's disease may also be associated with increased susceptibility to ankylosing spondylitis, even in the absence of B27, and even in the absence of clinical expression of psoriasis or inflammatory bowel disease[44,45,47,48]. Even 'primary' ankylosing spondylitis should be considered a clinical syndrome consisting of a heterogeneous group of phenotypically similar diseases with different genetic and non-genetic (environmental) predisposing factors[44]. Therefore, lack of an absolute epidemiological association between ankylosing spondylitis and B27 cannot be used as evidence for the existence of a linked distinct 'illness susceptibility' gene and against a direct functional role for B27 in the aetiopathogenesis of the disease.

If only a single gene other than B27 were responsible for all the cases of ankylosing spondylitis, one would expect the B27-positive and B27-negative patients to show an identical clinical picture as well as similar familial aggregation[11,44,45,47]. The present evidence, as discussed earlier, indicates that B27-negative patients less frequently get acute anterior uveitis and have a somewhat later age of onset of their disease than the B27-positive patients (Table 2.2).

## Heterogeneity of B27

In an attempt to ascertain why only a small minority of B27-positive individuals get ankylosing spondylitis and related disease, one needs to investigate the possibility that the B27 gene product observed in diseased individuals might be different from that of normal individuals. Karr *et al.*[70] failed to demonstrate any differences by isoelectric focusing (IEF) and peptide mapping between B27 antigens from healthy individuals and from patients with ankylosing spondylitis.

Recent studies have used monoclonal antibodies, cytotoxic T lymphocytes (CTL), and IEF gel analysis to probe genetic heterogeneity of B27[71-77]. Although B27 is one of the best-defined serological specificities, at least three CTL-defined subtypes of B27 have been recognized by alloreactive CTL and by B27-restricted virus-specific CTL. These subtypes have been designated as B27W, B27K, B27C and B27.1, B27.2 and B27.3, respectively[72-74,77]. They share a constant B27-M1 epitope determined by the use of monoclonal antibody B27-M1, but can be distinguished on the basis of their differential reactivity with another monoclonal antibody B27-M2. A fourth subtype, designated as B27D or B27.4, as well as other additional variants have now been discovered[75,76]. Choo et al.[75,76] have reported six variants of B27, detected by IEF get electrophoresis; these variants have been assigned lower-case letters, i.e. B27a, B27b, B27c, B27d, B27e and B27f. Correlations of all the known B27 variants by comparing iso-electric focusing patterns of B27 molecules immunoprecipitated from representative B27 variant cells have recently been reported by the same group of investigators[78,79]. The results are shown in Table 2.3. The IEF-defined variant B27a has been further divided into two subgroups (B27a.1 and B27a.2) on the basis of reactivity with a monoclonal antibody P56.1. It is worth noting that three IEF-defined variants (B27b, B27c and B27d) cannot be distinguished from each other by serological means. Thus, heterogeneity of B27 has been clearly demonstrated using monoclonal antibodies, CTL and IEF gel analysis, and in all eight different variants of B27 can now be distinguished (Table 2.4).

Vega et al.[72] have recently determined the amino acid sequence of B27.1 (B27a.1), the major subtype in Caucasians, B27.2 (B27e), as well as B27.3 (B27b), a subtype that is mostly seen in Oriental populations. There are only three amino acid substitutions between B27.1 and B27.2: aspartate-77, threonine-80, and leucine-81 in B27.1 are changed to asparagine-77, isoleucine-80, and alanine-81 in B27.2. HLA-B27.3 subtype has serine at position 77; thus residue 77 is different in all three subtypes. B27.3 differs from the other two subtypes in having glutamine instead of valine at position 152. Rojo et al.[74] have now clearly demonstrated, using antibodies against the chemically synthesized 63–84 peptide from B27.1, the contribution of the hypervariable region spanning residues 63 to 84 to the alloantigenic specificity of HLA-B27. The amino acid sequence of two additional variants of B27 has been studied (B27f and B27D) and all the five B27 subtypes so far studied differ by only 2 to 4 amino acid substitutions and the amino acids at positions 77 and 152 may determine the

TABLE 2.3 Serological reactivity of B27 variants

| B27 variants | Monoclonal antibody | | | | | Alloantiserum |
| | P7.1 | B27M1 | 145.2 | B27M2 | P56.1 | KC-MJA3 |
|---|---|---|---|---|---|---|
| B27a.1 (B27.1,B27W) | + | + | + | + | + | + |
| B27a.2 | + | + | + | + | − | + |
| B27b<br>B27c } \|(B27.3,B27C) | + | + | + | (W) | − | + |
| B27c | | | | | | |
| B27d | + | + | + | + | + | − |
| B27e (B27 2,B27K) | + | + | + | − | + | − |
| B27f | + | + | + | − | + | + |
| — (B27.4,B27D) | + | + | + | (W) | − | + |

W = weak reactivity.
Choo et al.[75 76 78]


TABLE 2.4 Comparison of known HLA-B27 variants

| CTL/IEF-defined | IEF-defined | CTL-defined |
|---|---|---|
| B27W | B27a | B27.1 |
| B27C | { B27b<br>B27c } | B27.3 |
| — | B27d | — |
| B27K | B27e | B27.2 |
| — | B27f | — |
| B27D | — | B27.4 |

Choo et al [75 76 78]


serological specificities recognized by monoclonal antibodies B27M2 and P56.1, respectively[78].

The prevalence of B27 subtype appears to vary in different populations, but no subtype has been found to be preferentially associated with ankylosing spondylitis. It has still not been possible to identify any single B27 epitope that is uniquely disease related[77,80,81]. The distribution of the various subtypes has been observed to be the same among Dutch spondylitis patients and healthy controls[77]. Studies by Choo et al. (personal communication) in California have also failed to reveal any difference. These observations raise the possibility that a public antigenic determinant shared by the various B27 subtypes, and not the private determinants may have a more direct role in the pathogenesis of ankylosing spondylitis[77]. Studies are in progress to determine those unique amino acid substitutions that are conserved among all the B27 subtypes because these amino acid sites may form the major antigenic epitope of B27 that may directly correlate with the disease at the molecular level. The structure of the carbohydrate moiety of B27 also needs to be studied since differences of this moiety could affect molecular function and be undetectable by allospecific sera because these sera are directed primarily against polypeptide structures. There are no significant differences in the expression of B27 antigen on mononuclear cells obtained from patients with ankylosing spondylitis and healthy controls[82].

Complete sequence of HLA-B27 cDNA has now been identified through determination of the sequence of an HLA-B27 mRNA[83]. The structure of the extracellular domains of the B27 molecule deduced from the observed nucleotide sequence was found to be virtually identical to the amino acid sequence recently reported by Ezquerra *et al.*[84]. Recently Coppin and McDevitt[81] have cloned three B27 genes from DNA of three different Epstein–Barr virus-transformed cell lines, one obtained from a normal individual, one from a patient suffering from ankylosing spondylitis and the third from a homozygous consanguinous cell line of unknown origin. The comparison of DNA sequences of HLA-B27 exons for $\alpha_1$, $\alpha_2$ and $\alpha_3$ domains from these three sources did not show any difference. However, this lack of any difference does not mean that B27 itself is not involved in the pathogenesis of the disease. It is, for example, still possible that B27 undergoes a structural modification as a result of interaction with an exterior microbial agent. Most likely, ankylosing spondylitis is caused by a multifactorial aetiology where B27 interacts with other genetic and environmental factors. There is a need to look also for non-HLA-linked disease predisposing genetic factors that may segregate in families with ankylosing spondylitis, as suggested by Brewerton *et al.*[85] The initial observation of a possible association of a specific phenotype, MZ, of $\alpha_1$-antitrypsin ($\alpha_1$-proteinase inhibitor) with ankylosing spondylitis and acute anterior uveitis[85] has not been confirmed by subsequent studies[85a]. The genetic determinants for

$\alpha_1$- antitrypsin, along with that for the Gm system, are found on chromosome 14, but no association has been found between specific Gm allotypes and ankylosing spondylitis[86,87]. The finding by Kijlstra et al.[88] of excess of Gm 1, 3, 17; 23; 5, 13, 21 phenotype in patients with associated anterior uveitis has also not been confirmed[85a].

## Possible role of *Klebsiella* in disease pathogenesis

Among the environmental factors triggering ankylosing spondylitis, infectious causes have long been suspected but never established. The knowledge that B27 is also associated with Reiter's syndrome and reactive arthritis following enteritis by certain gram-negative organisms such as *Yersinia*, *Shigella* and *Salmonella*, has led to a search for microbes that might trigger primary ankylosing spondylitis. Recent studies by two groups of investigators[42,52] have suggested a possible role for certain *Klebsiella* species in initiation of the disease process, but their interpretation of the role of these microbes differs widely.

Ebringer et al.[89] have noted that spondylitis patients show an increased prevalence of colonization of the gut by *Klebsiella* during episodes of active disease, and exhibit a specific elevation of serum IgA antibody to *Klebsiella* antigen. They have suggested that there may be a stereochemical resemblance between certain *Klebsiella* antigen(s) and B27, and that the antibody produced by the host against such cross-reacting epitopes on *Klebsiella* antigen(s) will also have an affinity for self-antigen(s) (molecular cross-reactivity hypothesis), and the disease results from tissue damage caused by such antibacterial antibodies binding to the cross-reacting self antigen(s).

Geczy et al.[68,90,91] have shown that antibodies raised in animals against certain strains of *Klebsiella* react very specifically with cells from about 80% of B27-positive patients with ankylosing spondylitis, but not with B27-positive cells from normal individuals. However, when B27-positive cells from normal individuals are exposed to the broth in which these *Klebsiella* organisms had been cultured, the cells show reactivity with the anti-*Klebsiella* antibodies; a similar modifying effect has not been observed with cells from B27-negative patients with ankylosing spondylitis. These investigators suggest that the absorption of a *Klebsiella*-derived factor onto B27 may be an important element in the pathogenesis of ankylosing spondylitis, and that the factor responsible for cross-reactivity may be generated by a bacterial plasmid.

Because of a lack of independent confirmation of the work of these two groups of investigators by many other researchers, a role for *Klebsiella* in primary ankylosing spondylitis has not yet gained global acceptance[68,92]. However, some recent observations seem to have heightened interest in *Klebsiella* and other enteric pathogens[91,93–94a]; further details will be given in a future volume in this series.

## HLA-B27 AS AN AID TO DIAGNOSIS

The frequency of B27 among Caucasian patients with ankylosing spondylitis is close to 92%, but the association with other spondyloarthropathies is relatively weaker, e.g. it is close to 75% in Reiter's syndrome[10,11,53,95]. Thus, the sensitivity of the B27 test is 92% for ankylosing spondylitis, and 75% for Reiter's syndrome[35,95,96]. Since 8% of the general population is B27-positive, the specificity of the B27 test for both of these diseases is 92% in whites. The frequency of B27 among other racial groups is shown in Table 2.1. Since B27 typing cannot be used as a perfect test for these diseases (it is not 100% sensitive and 100% specific), one cannot use it as a screening test because an overwhelming majority of the B27-positive individuals in the general population remain unaffected and spondylitis can occasionally occur in B27-negative individuals[35,95].

It needs to be emphasized that in the practice of medicine the history, physical examination, and laboratory investigation all serve the same purpose: they reduce the uncertainty of diagnosis to an acceptable level. A careful history and physical examination are an essential first step; an overwhelming majority of patients with ankylosing spondylitis can be readily diagnosed clinically on the basis of history, physical examination, and roentgenographic findings, and therefore do not need the B27 test[35,95]. However, the status of the sacroiliac joints on standard pelvic radiographs may not always be easy to interpret; some patients may present in an early phase of the disease with normal or equivocal roentgenographic findings; the earliest radiologic changes of sacroiliitis may be difficult to recognize with certainty in adolescents; and some rheumatological and non-rheumatological conditions may cause sacroiliac joint changes that are roentgenographically indistinguishable from those due to inflamm-ation[35]. Therefore, when a diagnosis of ankylosing spondylitis is clinically suspected in such circumstances where a patient exhibits clinical features suggestive but not diagnostic of the disease, detection of B27 further increases the probability that the presumptive diagnosis is correct[35,95].

In patients with back pain in whom ankylosing spondylitis is not suggested by either history or physical examination, B27 typing is inappropriate; a positive result would still not permit the diagnosis of ankylosing spondylitis to be made[35,95]. It cannot be overemphasized that the presence of B27 does not establish the diagnosis of any particular disease; it, like any other test, provides a probability state-ment on the existence of the disease in the patient. Conversely, the absence of B27 does not exclude these diseases, since all these diseases may occur in individuals who lack B27[35,95]. Moreover, since ankylosing spondylitis and related spondyloarthropathies all show an association with B27, the differentiation between these diseases is purely on a clinical basis. B27 typing, however, has become useful in clinical research for understanding the full spectrum of various forms of spondyloarthropathies[97,98]. B27 typing can also identify individuals at somewhat increased risk of developing spondyloarthropathies, but this is of no real clinical value at present since effective means of prevention are not currently available, and the majority of the B27-positive individuals never develop these diseases. The clinician must avoid inducing undue anxiety in healthy B27-positive individuals.

## ACKNOWLEDGEMENTS

This work was supported by a grant from the National Institute of Arthritis, Diabetes and Digestive and Kidney Diseases (Grant No. AM-20618 Northeast Ohio Multipurpose Arthritis Center). I am grateful to Kathy Kaltenbach and Nancy Kessler for excellent sec-retarial assistance.

References

1. Brewerton, D. A., Hart, F. D., Nicholls, A., *et al.* (1973). Ankylosing spondylitis and HL-A 27. *Lancet*, **1**, 904

2. Schlosstein, L., Terasaki, P. I., Bluestone, R., *et al.* (1973). High association of an HL-A antigen, W27, with ankylosing spondylitis. *N. Engl. J. Med.*, **288,** 704
3. Stastny, P. (1980). Rheumatoid arthritis. In Terasaki, P. I. (ed.) *Histocompatibility Testing 1980*, pp. 681–7. (Los Angeles: UCLA Tissue Typing Laboratory)
4. Payami, H., Thomson, G., Khan, M. A., Grennan, D. M., Sanders, P., Dyer, P. and Dostal, C. (1986). Genetics of rheumatoid arthritis. *Tissue Antigens*, **27,** 57–63
5. Dausett, J. (1981). The major histocompatibility complex in man. *Science*, **213,** 1469–74
6. Benacerraf, B. (1981). Role of MHC gene products in immune regulation. *Science*, **212,** 1229–38
7. McDevitt, H. O. (1986). The molecular basis of autoimmunity. *Clin. Res.*, **34,** 163–75
8. Strominger, J. L. (1986). Biology of the human histocompatibility leukocyte antigen (HLA) system and a hypothesis regarding the generation of autoimmune diseases. *J. Clin. Invest.*, **77,** 1411–15
9. Khan, M. A. (1985). Spondylarthropathies in non-Caucasian populations of the world. In Ziff, M. and Cohen, S. B. (eds.) *The Spondylarthropathies*, Vol. 9, pp. 91–9. (New York: Raven Press)
10. Tiwari, J. L. and Terasake, P. I. (1985). *HLA and Disease Associations*, pp. 85–100. (New York: Springer-Verlag)
11. Woodrow, J. C. (1977). Histocompatibility antigens and rheumatic diseases. *Semin. Arthritis Rheum.*, **6,** 257–76
12. Gofton, J. P., Robinson, H. S. and Trueman, G. E. (1966). Ankylosing spondylitis in a Canadian Indian population. *Ann. Rheum. Dis.*, **25,** 525–7
13. Gofton, J. P., Lawrence, J. S., Bennett, P. H. and Burch, T. A. (1966). Sacro-iliitis in eight populations. *Ann. Rheum. Dis.*, **25,** 528–33
14. Gofton, J. P., Bennett, P. H., Smythe, H. A. and Decker, J. L. (1972). Sacroiliitis and ankylosing spondylitis in North American Indians. *Ann. Rheum. Dis.*, **31,** 474–81
15. Gofton, J. P., Chalmers, A., Price, G. E. and Reeve, C. E. (1975). HL-A 27 and ankylosing spondylitis in B.C. Indians. *J. Rheumatol.*, **2,** 314–18
16. Gofton, J. P. (1980). Epidemiology, tissue type antigen and Bechterew's syndrome (ankylosing spondylitis) in various ethnical populations. *Scand. J. Rheumatol.*, **9** (Suppl. 32), 166–8
17. Ford, D. K., Henderson, E., Price, G. E. and Stein, H. B. (1977). Yersinia-related arthritis in the Pacific Northwest. *Arthritis Rheum.*, **20,** 1226–30
18. Kuberski, T. T., Morse, H. G., Rate, R. G. and Bonnell, M. D. (1983). Increased recovery of Klebsiella from the gastrointestinal tract of Reiter's syndrome and ankylosing spondylitis patients. *Br. J. Rheumatol.*, **22** (Suppl. 2), 85–90
19. Morse, H. G., Rate, R. G., Bonnell, M. D., *et al.* (1980). High frequency of HLA-B27 and Reiter's syndrome in Navajo Indians. *J. Rheumatol.*, **7,** 900–2
20. Muggia, A. L., Bennahum, D. A. and William, R. C., Jr (1971). Navajo arthritis – an unusual, acute, self-limited disease. *Arthritis Rheum.*, **14,** 348–55
21. Chalmers, I. M. (1980). Ankylosing spondylitis in African blacks. *Arthritis Rheum.*, **23,** 1366–70
22. Kalk, W. J., Maier, G., van Drimellen, M., Levin, J. and Reinach, S. G. (1983). HLA antigens and Graves' disease in Black South Africans. *Tissue Antigens.*, **2,** 7–15

23. Klemp, P., Meyers, O. L. and Du Toit, E. D. (1982). HLA-B27 and ankylosing spondylitis in African blacks. (Letter) *Arthritis Rheum.*, **25**, 716–17

24. Müller, A. S., Valkenburg, H. A., Greenwood, B. M. (1972). Rheumatoid arthritis in three West African populations. *East Afr. Med. J.*, **49**, 75–83

25. Payne, R., Feldman, M., Cann, H. and Bodmer, J. G. (1977). A comparison of HLA data in the North American black with African black and North American caucasoid populations. *Tissue Antigens*, **9**, 135–47

26. Ryder, L. P., Anderson, E., Svejgaard, A. (eds.) (1979). *HLA and Disease Registry: Third Report* (Copenhagen: Munksgaard)

27. Thomas, A. F., Solomon, L. and Rabson, A. (1975). Polyarthritis associated with *Yersinia enterocolitica* infection. *S. Afr. Med. J.*, **49**, 18–20

28. Khan, M. A., Braun, W. E., Kushner, I., Grecek, D. E., Muir, W. A. and Steinberg, A. G. (1977). HLA-B27 in ankylosing spondylitis: differences in frequency and relative risk in American Blacks and Caucasians. *J. Rheumatol.*, **4** (Suppl. 3), 39–43

29. Khan, M. A. (1984). Spondylarthropathies in non-Caucasians. In Calin, A. (ed.) *Spondylarthropathies*, pp. 265–77. (Orlando: Grune and Stratton)

30. Baum, J. and Ziff, M. (1971). The rarity of ankylosing spondylitis in the black race. *Arthritis Rheum.*, **14**, 12–18

31. van der Linden, S. M., Valkenburg, H. A. and Cats, A. (1985). Risk for development of ankylosing spondylitis in HLA-B27-positive individuals: consensus, conflicts and questions. In Ziff, M. and Cohen, S. B. (eds.) *The Spondylarthropathies*, Vol. 9, pp. 83–9. (New York: Raven Press)

32. Calin, A. (ed.) (1984). *Spondylarthropathies*. (Orlando: Grune and Stratton)

33. van der Linden, S. M. and Khan, M. A. (1984). The risk of ankylosing spondylitis in HLA-B27 positive individuals: A reappraisal. *J. Rheumatol.*, **11**, 727–8

34. van der Linden, S. M. and Khan, M. A. (1986). Letters to the Editor. *J. Rheumatol.*, **13**, 220–4

35. Khan, M. A. and Kushner, I. (1984). Diagnosis of ankylosing spondylitis. In A. S. Cohen (ed.) *Progress in Clinical Rheumatology*, Vol. 1, pp. 145–78. (Orlando: Grune and Stratton)

36. van der Linden, S., Valkenbert, H. A., de Jong, B. M., *et al.* (1984). The risk of developing ankylosing spondylitis in HLA-B27 positive individuals: a comparison of relatives of AS patients with the general population. *Arthritis Rheum.*, **3**, 241

37. Khan, M. A. (1987). Ankylosing spondylitis. In Calin, A. (ed.) *Spondylarthropathies*, pp. 69–117. (Orlando: Grune and Stratton)

38. van der Linden, J. M. J. P., DeCeulaer, K., van Romunde, L. K. J. and Cats, A. (1977). Ankylosing spondylitis without HLA-B27. *J. Rheumatol.*, **4** (Suppl. 3), 54–6

39. Khan, M. A., Kushner, I. and Braun, W. E. (1977). Comparison of clinical features in HLA-B27 positive and negative patients with ankylosing spondylitis. *Arthritis Rheum.*, **20**, 909–12

40. Nahir, M., Scharf, Y., Brik, R., Scharf, Y., Gidoni, O. and Barzilai, A. (1979). The influence of HLA-B27 on the clinical picture of ankylosing spondylitis. *Rheumatol. Rehabil.*, **18**, 10–12

41. Scharf, J., Nahir, M., Scharf, J., Brick, R., Gidoni, O., Barzilai, A. and Zonis, S. (1979). Anterior uveitis in ankylosing spondylitis: a histocompatibility study. *Ann. Ophthalmol.*, **11**, 1061–2

42. van der Linden, S., Valkenburg, H. A. and Cats, A. (1983). Is uveitis associated

with ankylosing spondylitis or with HLA-B27? *Br. J. Rheumatol.*, **22** (Suppl. 2), 146–7

43. Edmonds, J. P. and Bashir, H. V. (1978). Family studies in HLA B27 negative ankylosing spondylitis. *Aust. N.Z. J. Med.*, **8** (Suppl. 1), 179
44. Khan, M. A., Kushner, I. and Braun, W. E. (1980). Genetic heterogeneity in primary ankylosing spondylitis. *J. Rheumatol.*, **7**, 383–6
45. Hammoudeh, M. and Khan, M. A. (1983). Genetics of HLA associated diseases: Ankylosing spondylitis. *J. Rheumatol.*, **10**, 301
46. Khan, M. A., Kushner, I. and Braun, W. E. (1978). A subgroup of ankylosing spondylitis associated with HLA-B7 in American blacks. *Arthritis Rheum.*, **21**, 528–30
47. Woodrow, J. C. (1985). Genetic aspects of spondylarthropathies. *Clin. Rheum. Dis.*, **11**, 1
48. Gladman, D. D., Urowitz, M. B., Anhorn, K. A. B., Chalmers, A. and Mervart, H. (1986). Discordance between HLA-B27 and ankylosing spondylitis: A family investigation. *J. Rheumatol.*, **13**, 129–36
49. Arnett, F. C. Jr (1984). HLA and the spondylarthropathies. In Calin, A. (ed.) *Spondylarthropathies*, pp. 297–321. (New York: Grune and Stratton)
50. Arnett, F. C. Jr, Hochberg, M. C. and Bias, W. B. (1977). Cross-reactive HLA antigens in B27-negative Reiter's syndrome and sacroiliitis. *Johns Hopkins Med. J.*, **141**, 193–7
51. Joysey, V. C. and Wolf, E. (1978). HLA-A, -B and -C antigens, their serology and cross-reaction. *Br. Med. Bull.*, **34**, 217–22
52. Khan, M. A. (1983). B7-CREG and ankylosing spondylitis. *Br. J. Rheumatol.*, **22** (Suppl. 2), 129–33
53. Khan, M. A., Askari, A. D., Braun, W. E. and Aponte, C. J. (1979). Low association of HLA-B27 with Reiter's syndrome in blacks. *Ann. Intern. Med.*, **90**, 202–3
54. Khan, M. A., Kushner, I., Braun, W. E., Zachary, A. A. and Steinberg, A. G. (1978). HLA-B27 homozygosity in ankylosing spondylitis: relationship to risk and severity. *Tissue Antigens*, **11**, 434–8
55. Steinberg, A. G. (1980). (Letter to the Editor). *Tissue Antigens.*, **16**, 265
56. Cohen, T. (1976). Are homozygous for HLA-B27 more susceptible to ankylosing spondylitis? *N. Engl. J. Med.*, **295**, 342
57. Arnett, F. C., Schacter, B. Z. and Hochberg, M. (1977). Homozygosity for HLA-B27: Impact on rheumatic disease expression in two families. *Arthritis Rheum.*, **20**, 797–804
58. Spencer, D. G., Dick, H. M. and Dick, W. C. (1979). Ankylosing spondylitis – the role of HLA-B27 homozygosity. *Tissue Antigens.*, **14**, 379–84
59. Möller, P. and Berg, K. (1983). Family studies in Bechterew's syndrome (ankylosing spondylitis) III: Genetics. *Clin. Genet.*, **24**, 73–89
60. Suarez-Almazor, M. E. and Russell, A. S. (1986). B27 homozygosity and ankylosing spondylitis. (In press)
61. Khan, M. A., Kushner, I. and Braun, W. E. (1981). Association of HLA-A2 with uveitis in HLA-B27 positive patients with ankylosing spondylitis. *J. Rheumatol.*, **8**, 295–8
62. Kemple, K., Gatti, R. A., Leibold, W., Klinenberg, J. and Bluestone, R. (1979). HLA-D locus typing in ankylosing spondylitis and Reiter's syndrome. *Arthritis Rheum.*, **22**, 371–5

63. Dejelo, C. I., Braun, W. E., Khan, M. A. and Clough, J. D. (1978). HLA-DR antigens and ankylosing spondylitis. *Transplant Proc.*, **10**, 971–2
64. Braun, W. E., Dejelo, C. L., Clough, J. D., Beck, K. A., Schacter, B. Z. and Khan, M. A. (1978). No association of known DR antigens with ankylosing spondylitis. *N. Engl. J. Med.*, **298**, 744–5
65. Raffoux, C., Faure, G., Netter, P., Streiff, F., Pourell, J. and Gaucher, A. (1978). No association of known DRw antigens with ankylosing spondylitis. *Arthritis Rheum.*, **21**, 977
66. Khan, M. A. and Skosey, J. L. (1987). Ankylosing spondylitis and associated diseases. In Max Samter (ed.) *Immunologic Diseases*. 4th Edn. (Boston: Little, Brown)
67. Ziff, M. and Cohen, S. B. (eds.) (1985). Advances in inflammation research, Vol. 9.*The Spondyloarthropathies*. (New York: Raven Press)
68. Keat, A. C. (1983). Reiter's syndrome and reactive arthritis in perspective. *N. Engl. J. Med.*, **309**, 1606
69. Kellegren, J. H. (1962). Diagnostic criteria for population studies. *Bull. Rheum. Dis.*, **13**, 291
70. Karr, R. W., Hahn, Y. and Schwartz, B. D. (1982). Structural identity of human histocompatibility leukocyte antigen-B27 molecule from patients with ankylosing spondylitis and normal individuals. *J. Clin. Invest.*, **69**, 443
71. Kaneoka, H., Engleman, E. G. and Grumet, F. C. (1983). Immunochemical variants of HLA-B27. *J. Immunol.*, **130**, 1288
72. Vega, M. A., Ezquerra, A., Rojo, S., Aparicio, P., Bragado, R., De Castro, J. L. A. (1985). Structural analysis of an HLA-B27 functional variant: Identification of residues that contribute to the specificity of recognition by cytolytic T lymphocytes. *Proc. Natl. Acad. Sci, USA.*, **82**, 7394–8
73. Vega, M. A., Wallace, L., Rojo, S., Bragado, R., Aparicio, P. and Lopez de Castro, J. A. (1985). Delineation of functional sites in HLA-B27 antigens: Molecular analysis of HLA-B27 variant wewak I defined by cytolytic T lymphocytes. *J. Immunol.*, **135**, 3323–32
74. Rojo, S., Lopez de Castro, J. A., Aparicio, P., van Seventer, G. and Bragado, R. (1986). HLA-B27 antigenicity: antibodies against the chemically synthesized 63-84 peptide from HLA-B27.1 display alloantigenic specificity and discriminate among HLA-B27 subtypes. *J. Immunol.*, **137**, 904–10
75. Choo, S. Y., Seyfreid, C., Hansen, J. A. and Nepom, G. T. (1986). Tryptic peptide mapping identifies structural heterogeneity among six variants of HLA-B27. *Immunogenetics*, **23**, 409–12
76. Choo, S. Y., Antonelli, P., Nisperos, B., Nepom, G. T. and Hansen, J. A. (1986). Six variants of HLA-B27 identified by isoelectric focusing. *Immunogenetics*, **23**, 24–9
77. Breur-Vriesendorp, B. S., Huis, B., Dekker, A. J., Breuning, M. H. and Ivanyi, P. (1985). Subtypes of antigen HLA-B27 (B27W and B27K) defined by cytotoxic T lymphocytes: Identification of a third subtype (B27C) prevalent in Oriental populations. In Ziff, M. and Cohen, S. B. (eds.) *The Spondyloarthropathies*, pp. 55–6. (New York: Raven Press)
78. Choo, S. Y., Rojo, S., Lopez de Castro, J. A. and Hansen, J. A. (1986). Primary structural differences in HLA-B27 variants: Implication for mapping serologic determinants. *Human Immunol.*, **17**, 163
79. Beatty, P. G., Fan, L., Nelson, K., Choo, S. Y. and Hansen, J. A. (1986). HLA-

B27 epitopes defined by monoclonal antibodies and cloned cytotoxic T lymphocytes. *Human Immunol.*, **17**, 162–3

80. Turek, P. J., Grumet, F. C. and Engleman, E. G. (1985). Molecular variants of the HLA-B27 antigen in healthy individuals and patients with spondyloarthropathies. *Immunol. Rev.*, **86**, 71

81. Coppin, H. L., and McDevitt, H. O. (1986). Absence of polymorphism between HLA-B27 genomic exon sequences isolated from normal donors and ankylosing spondylitis patients. *J. Immunol.*, **137**, 2168–72

82. Van Der Gaag, R., Luyenduk, L., Linssen, A. and Kijlstra, A. (1985). Expression of HLA-B27 antigens on mononuclear lymphocytes in ankylosing spondylitis. *Clin. Exp. Immunol.*, **60**, 311–15

83. Szöts, H., Riethmüller, G., Weiss, E. and Meo, T. (1986). Complete sequence of HLA-B27 cDNA identified through the characterization of structural markers unique to the HLA-A, -B, and -C allelic series. *Proc. Natl. Acad. Sci. USA.*, **83**, 1428–32

84. Ezquerra, A., Bragado, R., Vega, M. A., Strominger, J. L., Woody, J. and Lopez de Castro, J. A. (1985). Primary structure of papain-solubilized human histocompatibility antigen HLA-B27. *Biochemistry*, **24**, 1733–41

85. Brewerton, D. A., Webley, M. and Ward, A. M. (1985). Acute anterior uveitis and the fourteenth chromosome. In Ziff, M. and Cohen, S. B. (eds.) *The Spondyloarthropathies*, pp. 225–9. (New York: Raven Press)

85a. Derhagg, P. J. F. M., Feltkamp, T. E. W., Broekema, N. *et al.* (1986). HLA-B27 and other genetic markers in patients with AAU and AS. (Abstract). Presented at EULAR Symposium, Rome, October 16–18, 1986. p. 37

86. Gran, J. T., Gaardner, P. I. and Husby, G. (1985). IgG heavy chain (Gm) allotypes in ankylosing spondylitis. *Clin. Rheumatol.*, **4**, 73

87. Russell, A. S. and Pandey, J. P. (1986). Immunoglobulin allotypes in patients with B27 positive ankylosing spondylitis. *J. Rheumatol.*, **12**, 1200

88. Kijlstra, A., Linssen, A. and Ockhuizen, T. (1984). Association of Gm allotypes with the occurrence of ankylosing spondylitis in HLA-B27-positive anterior uveitis. *Am. J. Ophthalmol.*, **98**, 732

89. Ebringer, A., Baines, M. and Ptaszynska, T. (1985). Spondyloarthritis, uveitis HLA-B27 and Klebsiella. *Immunol. Rev.*, **86**, 101

90. Geczy, A. F., Prendergast, J. K., Sullivan, J. S., Upfold, L. I., Edmonds, J. P. and Bashir, H. V. (1985). Possible role of enteric organisms in the pathogenesis of the seronegative arthropathies. In Ziff, M. and Cohen, S. B. (eds.) *The Spondyloarthropathies*, pp. 129–37. (New York: Raven Press)

91. McGuigan, L. E., Geczy, A. F., Prendergast, J. K., Edmonds, J. P., Hart, H. H. and Bashir, H. V. (1986). HLA-B27 associated cross-reactive marker on the cells of New Zealand patients with ankylosing spondylitis. *Ann. Rheum. Dis.*, **45**, 144

92. Kinsella, T. D. (1985). Review of research on the role of Klebsiella antigens in the spondylarthropathies. In Ziff, M. and Cohen, S. B. (eds.) *The Spondyloarthropathies*, pp. 139–47. (New York: Raven Press)

93. van Bohemen, C. G., Nabbe, A. J. J. B. M., Decker-Saeys, A. J., *et al.* (1985). Antibodies to enterobacterial cell envelope antigens in ankylosing spondylitis. In Ziff, M. and Cohen, S. B. (eds.) *The Spondyloarthropathies*, pp. 129–37. (New York: Raven Press)

94. van Rood, J. J., van Leeuwen, A., Ivanyi, P., Cats, A., *et al.* (1985). Blind confirmation of Geczy factor in ankylosing spondylitis. *Lancet.*, **2**, 943

94a. Schwimmbeck, P. L., Yu, D. T. Y. and Oldstone, M. B. A. (1987). Autoimmune pathogenesis for ankylosing spondylitis (AS) and Reiter's syndrome (RS): auto-antibodies against an epitope shared by HLA-B27 and Klebsiella in sera of HLA-B27 patients with AS and RS. *Clin. Res.*, **35**, 664A

95. Khan, M. A. and Khan, M. K. (1982). Diagnostic value of HLA-B27 testing in ankylosing spondylitis and Reiter's syndrome. *Ann. Intern. Med.*, **96**, 70

96. Khan, M. A. (1980). Clinical application of the HLA-B27 test in rheumatic disease: a current perspective. *Arch. Intern. Med.*, **140**, 177–80

97. Khan M. A., van der Linden, S., Kushner, I., *et al.* (1985). Spondylitic disease without evidence of sacroiliitis in relatives of HLA B27-positive ankylosing spondylitis patients. *Arthritis Rheum.*, **28**, 40

98. Lionarons, R. J., Van Zoeren, M., Verhagen, J. N. and Lammers, H. A. (1986). HLA-B27 associated reactive spondyloarthropathies in a Dutch military hospital. *Ann. Rheum. Dis.*, **45**, 141

# 3
# ANKYLOSING SPONDYLITIS: EARLY DIAGNOSIS BASED ON THE NATURAL HISTORY

*J. J. CALABRO*

## INTRODUCTION

The rheumatic diseases comprise well over 100 distinct entities affecting as many as 36 million Americans. Ankylosing spondylitis (AS) affects 3 million Americans and is third in frequency only to osteo-arthritis (16 million) and rheumatoid arthritis (6.5 million)[1]. In England, it has been estimated that there are at least 50 000 patients with AS, a prevalence comparable to that of gout[2].

In recent years, there has been enormous progress in our understanding of AS. In fact, it has emerged from a disorder of relative obscurity to one of considerable fascination and complexity equal in academic status to rheumatoid arthritis (RA) and systemic lupus erythematosus. Scientists from many disciplines have contributed to this expanding growth of knowledge including geneticists, immunologists, epidemiologists, pathologists, bacteriologists, biologists, and clinicians[2-7]. A great deal of this progress has been published in comprehensive reviews, including a multi-authored textbook on AS edited by Moll[2], a monograph by Wright and Moll[3], two monographs by Calin and associates[4,5] and proceedings from two international symposia on AS[6,7].

AS is a heterogeneous rheumatic disorder characterized by inflammation of the sacroiliac, spinal (axial), and large peripheral joints as

45

well as a host of systemic manifestations. Comprehensive management is clearly enhanced by early diagnosis and patient education, each of which depend in large measure on an understanding of the terminology, classification, epidemiology, pathogenesis, and natural history of AS.

## TERMINOLOGY AND CLASSIFICATION

### Terminology

The many terms used for AS have led to considerable confusion over the years[8–12]. Ankylosing spondylitis, the currently preferred term, was first introduced by Buckley in 1935[12]. Others include Marie–Strümpell disease, pelvospondylitis ossificans, Bechterew's syndrome, spondyloarthritis ankylopoietica, spondylitis deformans, and rheumatoid spondylitis. The last term, coined by the American Rheumatism Association (ARA), was finally abandoned and with good reason. It implied that AS was a variant of RA, but as shown in Table 3.1, there are notable differences between the two disorders[8,13]. Consequently, in 1964, the ARA reclassified AS as a distinct clinical entity apart from RA[14].

### Classification

AS is the prototype of the seronegative spondyloarthropathies which also include: (1) enteric arthritis or the arthritis of chronic inflammatory bowel disease (ulcerative colitis and regional enteritis), (2) psoriatic arthritis, and (3) Reiter's syndrome, including reactive arthritis due to enteric pathogens[15]. It is now widely acknowledged that these disorders are unified by a number of common features (Table 3.2)[1–27]. Moreover, they have little in common with RA, although they may occasionally mimic it, particularly in their initial presentations. Consequently, the former designation of these disorders as 'rheumatoid variants' should be abandoned[1,24].

'Spondarthritis' was a term introduced by Moll and colleagues in a 1974 publication[26]. The concept was developed further in 1976 by Wright and Moll in their monograph entitled *Seronegative Polyarthritis*[3]. As pointed out by Wright[27] in Moll's 1980 text on ankylosing

46

TABLE 3.1 Major differences between ankylosing spondylitis and rheumatoid arthritis

| Feature | Ankylosing spondylitis | Rheumatoid arthritis |
| --- | --- | --- |
| Ratio (men:women) | 3:1 | 1:3 |
| Sacroiliac joints | Early, symmetric changes except when only peripheral joints are initially involved* | Late, asymmetric changes noted in less than one-fourth of patients |
| Spinal (axial) joints | Regularly involved | Cervical spine often involved; dorsal and lumbar spine usually unaffected |
| Costovertebral joints | Early, diffuse involvement | Not involved |
| Peripheral joints | Initial presentation in up to 30% of patients; often asymmetric, primarily of lower limb joints | Invariably involved; usually symmetric including hands and feet as well as large joints |
| Recurrent acute anterior uveitis | Occurs in 30% of patients | No increased frequency |
| Rheumatoid nodules | Extremely rare | Present in 20% of patients |
| IgM Rheumatoid factor† | No increased frequency | Detectable in up to 85% of adults but in only 5% of juvenile-onset patients |
| HLA-B27 antigen | Present in up to 96% of patients | No increased frequency (same as general population) |

*Peripheral arthritis, particularly in children and women, may antedate back complaints by several years.
†By the latex fixation test, positive titre of 1 160 or greater

spondylitis[2], Calin and Fries misquoted the term 'spondylarthritides' as 'spondylarthritis' in their 1978 monograph on the subject[5]. Since then, common usage has resulted in widespread acceptance of the terms 'spondylarthritis', 'spondylarthopathy' and even 'spondyloarthropathy'[8].

TABLE 3.2 Unifying features of the seronegative spondyloarthropathies

---

Negative tests for IgM rheumatoid factor (latex fixation) and antinuclear antibodies

Absence of subcutaneous (rheumatoid) nodules

Inflammatory peripheral arthritis, often asymmetric

Roentgenographic evidence of sacroiliitis, with or without spondylitis

Overlap of mucocutaneous, ocular, genital, and gastrointestinal manifestations

High frequency of enthesopathy, characterized clinically by heel pain or other localized tender areas from inflammation of ligaments, tendons, or fascia, and roentgenographically by osseous proliferation and/or erosions at these sites

Tendency to cluster in families

Striking association with the inherited antigen HLA-B27

---

## EPIDEMIOLOGY AND PATHOGENESIS

### Genetic predisposition

The initial disclosure and subsequent world-wide confirmation of an unusually high frequency of the inherited antigen HLA-B27 in both patients and first-degree relatives provides overwhelming evidence of a genetic predisposition in the pathogenesis of AS[28–30]. Historically, these observations were first reported almost simultaneously in 1973 from both London and Los Angeles. In the London survey[28], B27 was identified in 96% of 75 patients with AS, in 50% of 60 first-degree relatives, but in only 4% of 75 controls. From Los Angeles[29], the antigen was detected in 88% of 40 patients with AS but in only 8% of 906 healthy controls, in 8% of 119 patients with RA, and in 9% of 66 patients with gout.

### Exogenous factors

Recent reports suggest that environmental or exogenous factors are also operative in the pathogenesis of AS[21,27,31–34]. Of particular relevance are reports in which the activity or flares of AS can be closely correlated with the presence of *Klebsiella pneumoniae* in stool cultures[35,36]. In fact, molecular mimicry between *Klebsiella* and the HLA-B27 antigen has been postulated[36], although this concept of cross-reactivity may be restricted to only certain strains of *Klebsiella*. However, a more recent study of antibodies to Enterobacteriaceae could find no difference between AS patients and controls[37].

## Prevalence

AS is the third most common form of chronic arthritis in the United States, affecting as many as 3 million Americans[38]. However, estimates of the prevalence of AS vary widely throughout the world, being directly proportional to the frequency with which the B27 antigen occurs in a given population[39,40]. Moreover, the frequency of subjects possessing the B27 antigen who will eventually develop AS remains unsettled. Based on two American surveys, one of B27-positive blood donors[38,41] and another of B27-positive tissue donors[42], it has been calculated that AS will develop in as many as 20% of both men and women harbouring the antigen.

## Associated disorders

In addition to AS, B27-positive subjects are also prone to develop recurrent attacks of acute anterior uveitis (without arthritis or spondylitis)[43-45] as well as Reiter's syndrome[40]. They are also predisposed to psoriatic arthritis and psoriatic spondylitis, although the correlation of B27 to these latter disorders is considerably less striking than with AS and Reiter's syndrome[40].

The frequent association between spondylitis and seemingly unrelated disorders, such as psoriasis, ulcerative colitis, and regional enteritis, has until recently defied explanation[27]. It now appears that among these disorders, the patients who are most apt to develop spondylitis are those positive for the B27 antigen. In fact, it has been estimated that the risk for developing spondylitis (i.e. enteric spondylitis) is 40 times greater in ulcerative colitis patients having the B27 than in those without the antigen[17].

## NATURAL HISTORY

The early diagnosis of AS rests on the recognition of three distinct modes of onset (back pain, peripheral arthritis, uveitis)[46]. The sub-

49

sequent course of disease is highly variable and unpredictable, as is the occurrence of systemic manifestations.

AS affects three times more men than women and begins most often in the prime of life, between the ages of 20 and 40[32,47]. Consequently, the condition occurs primarily in young men. Only 5–10% of cases begin in childhood, while the remaining 10–20% begin after the age of 40[47,48].

Modes of onset

Most patients present with back pain, usually of the lumbar spine and sacroiliac joints, but occasionally of the cervical or thoracic spine (Table 3.3). However, in approximately one-third of cases, most of whom are primarily children or women, disease begins in peripheral joints, often asymmetrically and usually of hips, knees, ankles and heels. Recurrent attacks of acute anterior uveitis are the sole presenting manifestation in about 2% of cases[46,47,49].

Early systemic signs may include fatigue, anorexia, weight loss, anaemia, acute anterior uveitis, and fever[13]. The febrile pattern is

TABLE 3.3  Modes of onset in ankylosing spondylitis*

| Modes of onset | Percentage of patients |
|---|---|
| Back Pain | 60 |
| Lumbosacral | 52 |
| Thoracic | 2 |
| Cervical | 6 |
| Peripheral Arthritis | 38 |
| Hip | 17 |
| Knee | 12 |
| Shoulder | 4 |
| Heel | 2 |
| Hand | 1 |
| Elbow | 1 |
| Ankle | 1 |
| Acute Anterior Uveitis | 2 |

*Based on a survey of 100 patients, consecutive referrals to an arthritis clinic.

typically intermittent (quotidian) with a daily rise and fall to normal. Although the fever is usually low grade, it may be high, especially in children, reaching levels of 40.5°C (105°F)[13,50]. In fact, patients with AS may even present as hyperpyrexia of undetermined origin[50]. Weight loss of more than 20 pounds is uncommon, although three patients with losses up to 50 and 100 pounds have been reported[13].

Course of disease

Whatever the mode of onset, recurrent or persistent back pain that is often nocturnal and of varying intensity is an eventual complaint, as is early morning stiffness that is characteristically relieved by activity. Patients will automatically ease back pain and paraspinal muscle spasm by adopting a flexed or bent-over posture. Diffuse costo-vertebral involvement also occurs early. Consequently, in the un-treated patient, some degree of kyphosis and diminished chest expansion are common sequelae. The usual course of AS is char-acterized by remissions and exacerbations that may be mild in some and severe in others. Rarely is the course persistently progressive, resulting in early and severe disability.

Peripheral arthritis occurs frequently in the course of AS[48,51]. While it is often transient and recurrent, it may become chronic in as many as 25% of patients[48]. Unlike RA, the peripheral arthritis of AS is usually asymmetric, affecting only one or a few large joints, such as hips, knees, or shoulders. Only rarely are the small joints of the hand and foot involved. Radiological features of AS that may aid in differentiation from RA include asymmetry, lack of demineralization, smaller erosions, propensity for bony ankylosis, and marginal peri-ostitis[51].

Symptomatic hip involvement may occur either early[52] or late[53] in the course of disease. However, patients with juvenile onset usually develop hip symptoms early[53]. Osteitis pubis, with erosive and sclerotic changes on roentgenographic examination, is frequently associated with AS[54]. Other joints affected include the sternoclavicular[55], tem-poromandibular[56,57] and cricoarytenoid[58,59]. Heel lesions are common in AS[60-62] whereas the tarsal tunnel syndrome is a rare manifestation[63]. For soft tissue lesions such as achillotendinitis, achillobursitis and plantar fasciitis, xeroradiography permits better confirmation than does conventional radiography[62].

## SYSTEMIC MANIFESTATIONS

Except for anterior uveitis which is more apt to occur in B27-positive patients, the frequency of systemic manifestations is comparable in patients with or without the B27 antigen[64]. Moreover, systemic manifestations occur regardless of whether the spondylitis is primary or secondary to Reiter's syndrome, ulcerative colitis, regional enteritis, or psoriasis[65]. Consequently, all patients should be monitored for ophthalmological, neurological, cardiovascular, or pulmonary involvement, since these comprise the major extra-articular manifestations observed in AS[24,65,66].

### Anterior uveitis (iridocyclitis)

While acute anterior uveitis is an uncommon presentation of AS, it eventually affects a third of patients (Figure 3.1)[65]. Patients should be cautioned that a tender and painful red eye with photophobia and lacrimation are ocular manifestations of AS and should be reported promptly to an ophthalmologist for appropriate evaluation and therapy. Attacks of uveitis are usually short-lived, subsiding within a few weeks, but recurrences are common. Rarely are attacks severe or protracted so as to cause loss of vision[65].

### Neurological manifestations

Neurological signs and symptoms may result from compression radiculitis or sciatica[67,68], from cord damage due to vertebral fracture or subluxation[68-71], or from the cauda equina syndrome[72-74]. The latter syndrome is characterized by bladder and rectal incontinence and saddle anaesthesia, usually occurring late in the course of disease and often leading to unnecessary prostatic surgery[65,73]. Other signs and symptoms include pain, numbness, or weakness of the lower limbs, impotency, and absence of ankle jerks[72].

The cauda equina syndrome is confirmed by characteristic myelographic abnormalities including posterior lumbar diverticula that may be missed unless myelography is performed with the patient in the

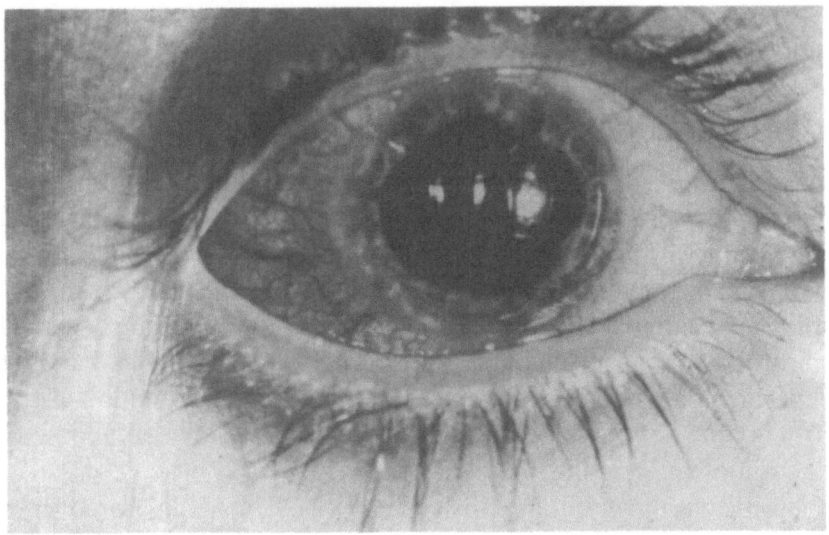

FIGURE 3.1 Anterior uveitis (iridocyclitis) is characterized by ciliary injection and irregularity of the pupil. Adhesions (synechiae) are present between the iris and lens at the 1 and 4 o'clock positions

supine position[75]. There is no effective therapy for the cauda equina syndrome. Limited trials with either corticosteroid therapy or laminectomy had no effect on the course of this slowly progressive neurological process[73].

## Cardiovascular findings

Abnormalities of the cardiovascular system include cardiomegaly, angina, pericarditis, conduction disturbances, and both aortic and mitral insufficiency[76–82].

In 97 patients with long-standing spondylitis, cardiovascular problems were found in 14%[77]. Of these 14 patients, eight had isolated aortic insufficiency, three isolated heart block, two combined aortic insufficiency and heart block, and one mitral insufficiency. Occasionally, cardiovascular lesions may antedate joint complaints[77,78] but may also regress spontaneously[77]. Cardiac conduction disturbances and aortic insufficiency are the most common cardiovascular manifestations[65]. Complete heart block with Stokes-Adams attacks are rare[81,82]. In fact, conduction defects rarely cause symptoms and are usually disclosed on routine electro- or echocardiography[76].

## Thoracopulmonary features

Involvement of the thorax is one of the essential features which differentiates AS from RA[83]. Rigidity of the chest cage is due primarily to involvement of the costovertebral joints. With advancing thoracic rigidity, respiratory movement becomes progressively restricted until respiration is almost entirely diaphragmatic. Chest pain that is usually inspiratory as well as dyspnoea on exertion rarely results, even with severe chest cage restriction. However, on pulmonary function testing, most patients have significant restriction of ventilatory excursion and reduction of lung volume[83,84].

Pleuritis with or without effusion may occur in AS[85]. Moreover, an uncommon pulmonary manifestation consists of apical or upper lobe fibrosis that occurs late in the course of disease[86–89]. Pulmonary fibrosis may progress to cavitation that may be mistaken for tuberculosis. Moreover, cavitary lesions are prone to intercurrent infection with *Aspergillus*[85,88,89], which may be treated successfully with transthoracic intracavitary instillation of antifungal agents[89].

## EARLY DIAGNOSIS

AS continues to remain one of the most commonly overlooked causes of back complaints in young people. Yet, all that is required for early diagnosis is the usual approach of all primary physicians – a complete history, including that of the family, and physical examination, as well as a critical interpretation of pertinent laboratory and roent-genographic findings[25].

## History and physical examination

If a patient complains of back pain there are several clues in the history that point to AS: (1) the back pain is insidious in onset, usually occurring in a patient younger than 40 years of age; (2) the back pain has persisted for at least three months; (3) the pain is intermittent, often worse at night; and (4) the pain is associated with early morning stiffness that improves with movement or exercise[90]. These historical

TABLE 3.4   Clinical tests for early detection of ankylosing spondylitis

| Test | Method | Interpretation |
|---|---|---|
| Sacroiliac compression | Exert direct compression over sacroiliac joints | Local tenderness suggests sacroiliac involvement which can be asymptomatic initially |
| Chest expansion | Measure maximum chest expansion at nipple line | Expansion of less than 3 cm is a clue to early costovertebal involvement |
| Fingers to floor | Patient bends forward with knees extended; distance in cm from fingertips to floor is measured | Inability to touch close to floor is evidence of early lumbar involvement |
| Schober test | Make a mark on the spine at the level of the iliac crests and then another 10 cm directly above while patient is standing upright. Patient then bends forward maximally and the distance between the two marks is measured | An increase of 3 cm or less indicates loss of lumbar flexion |
| Occiput to wall | Patient places heels and back against wall and tries to touch the wall with the back of the head without raising the chin above carrying level | Inability to touch head to wall signifies loss of cervical extension |

clues are highly sensitive and specific, especially useful in early diagnosis when clinical signs are minimal and X-ray findings are normal or equivocal.

On examination, certain simple tests will disclose typical abnormalities at an early stage (Table 3.4). For example, to unmask local tenderness from sacroiliitis, compress the sacroiliac joints bilaterally (Figure 3.2). In a surprising number of cases, the patient will not previously have reported pain specifically in the sacroiliac joints. To

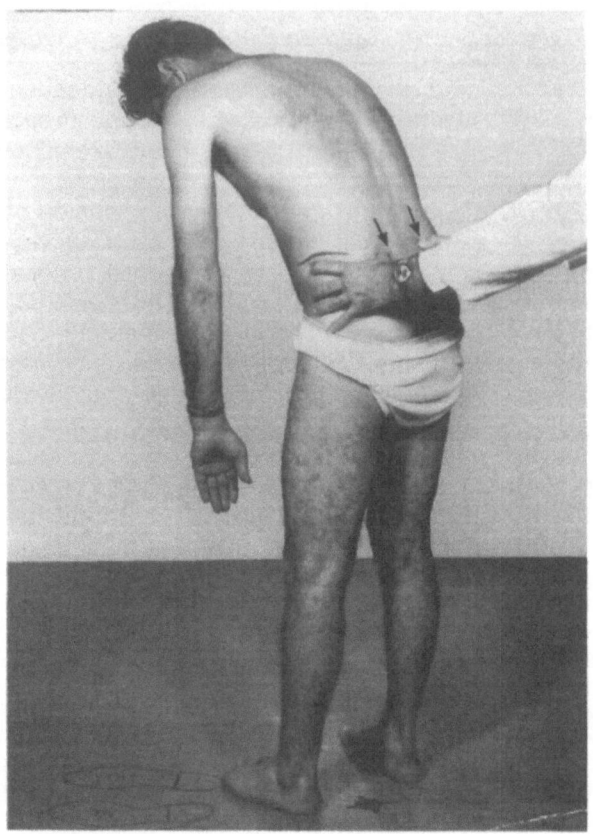

FIGURE 3.2    Direct compression is applied to the sacroiliac joints. Local tenderness or gluteal pain will reveal sacroiliitis, which is occasionally asymptomatic early

check for early costovertebral involvement that is frequently asymptomatic, measure the patient's chest expansion (Figure 3.3). If maximum expansion is less than 3 cm, your suspicions for AS should be aroused since normal chest expansion is 6 cm or greater.

   To check for lumbar involvement, ask the patient to touch to the floor while keeping the knees fully extended (Figure 3.4). Most patients are unable to reach with their fingertips much below knee level. Moreover, on examination of the lumbar spine, the normal lumbar lordosis may be lost because of paraspinal muscle spasm. One final

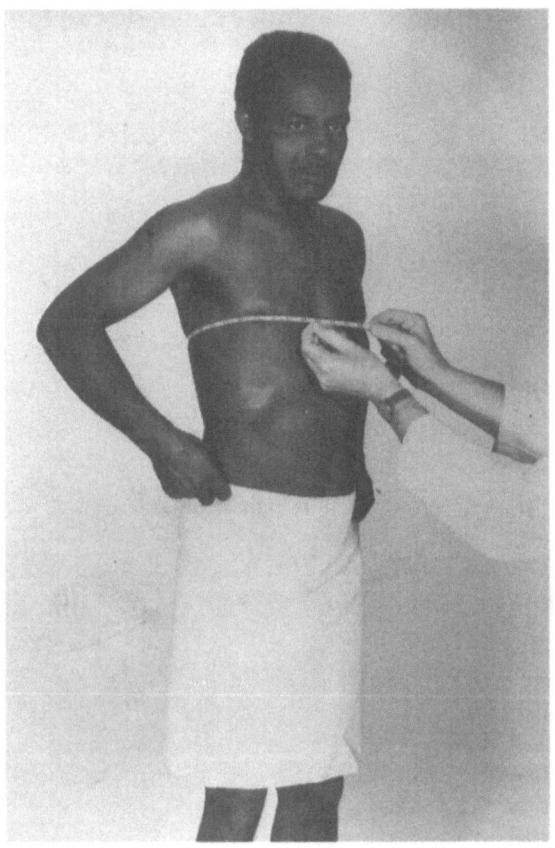

FIGURE 3.3  A simple test for detection of asymptomatic costovertebral involvement is to measure chest-cage expansion at the nipple line before and after deep inspiration. In ankylosing spondylitis, chest expansion is often 3 cm or less; normal expansion is 6 cm or greater

clue to early lumbar involvement is the Schober test (Figure 5A,B). If the measurement is less than 3 cm, the lumbar spine is affected.

Loss of cervical rotation and lateral bending, each of which are normally 45° to the right and 45° to the left, constitute early clues to cervical spine involvement, as does the occiput to wall test (Table 3.4). The inability to touch the head to the wall, measured in cm, signifies loss of cervical extension. With appropriate exercises, abnormal measurements may improve or revert to normal. Consequently, in

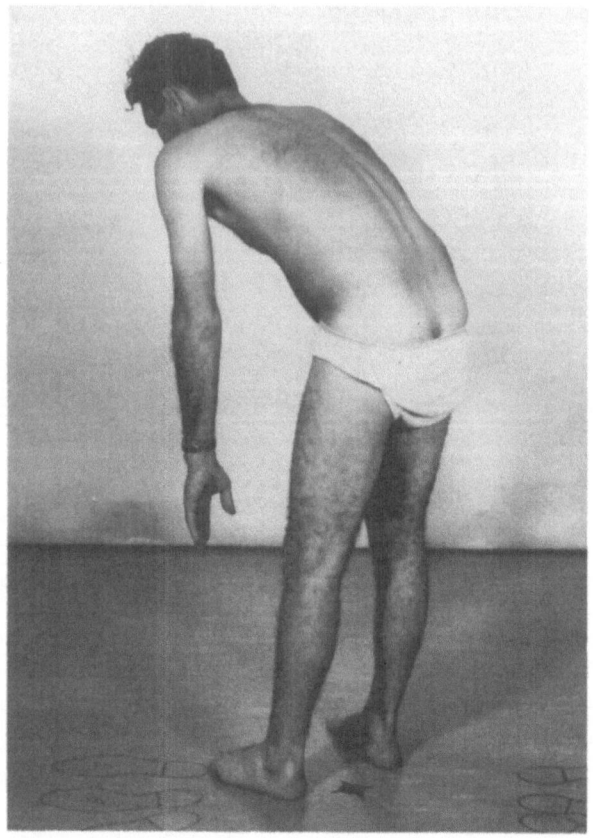

FIGURE 3.4    Limited spine flexion, disclosed by the fingers to floor test, is an early sign of lumbar spine involvement. When asked to touch the floor with the fingertips, while keeping knees extended, this 26-year-old man with back pain of 3 month's duration could bend only far enough to reach knee level

long-term management, these tests should become a routine part of the patient's evaluation at each follow up visit.

Early recognition of AS is difficult only when symptoms are limited either to peripheral joints or to recurrent anterior uveitis. Nevertheless, the physician should be aware that the early peripheral arthritis of AS primarily affects the lower limb joints, rather than the hands and wrists, the joints usually involved in RA.

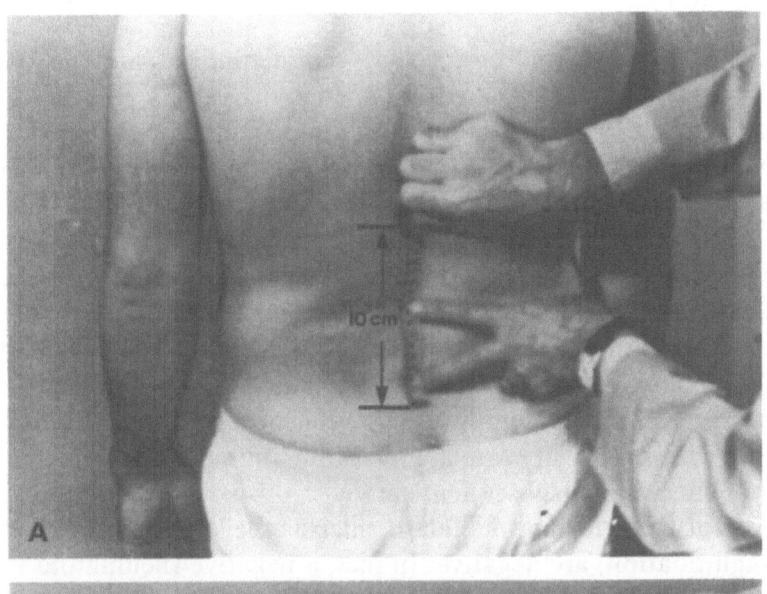

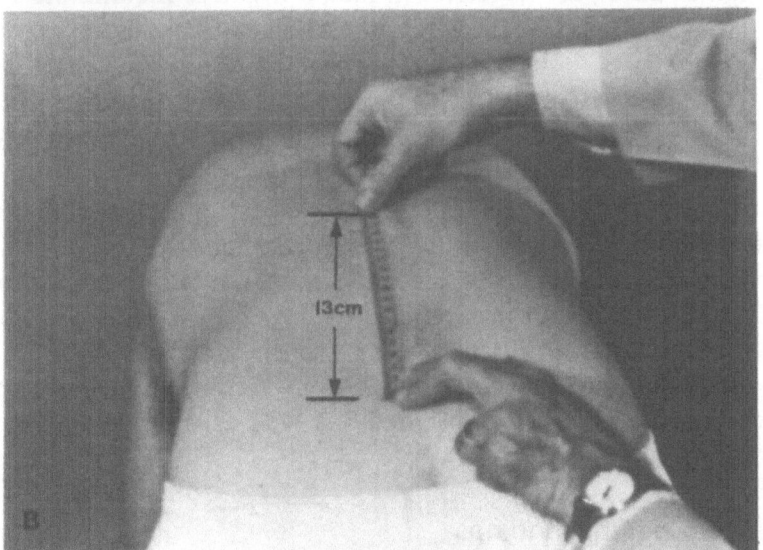

FIGURE 3.5   A, With the patient standing upright, the initial steps of the Schober test include placing a mark over the spine at the level of the iliac crests (L5/S1) and then, using a flexible tape, placing another mark 10 cm higher. B, Patient then bends forward maximally, keeping knees extended, and the distance between the two marks is measured. An increase of 3 cm or less between the two marks indicates loss of lumbar flexion

## Laboratory clues

When AS is active, the erythrocyte sedimentation rate (ESR) and serum IgA levels are elevated in most patients, as are other acute phase reactants[91,92]. Other laboratory abnormalities that occasionally occur include a minimal neutrophilic leukocytosis, low-grade anaemia, and a modest thrombocytosis (platelet count greater than $400\,000/\mu l$). Elevation of the serum iron, alkaline phosphatase, or creatinine phosphokinase have also been reported[91–94]. Except for febrile proteinuria, routine urinalysis is usually normal in AS. The subsequent development of proteinuria, however, may be a warning sign of evolving secondary amyloidosis or toxicity from drugs. An increase in the cerebrospinal fluid protein level has been observed in up to 40% of patients with AS[95,96]. It correlated with the presence of sciatica in one report[95] but not in a subsequent survey[96].

Tests for IgM rheumatoid factor, such as the latex fixation or sheep cell agglutination, are negative. In fact, a negative rheumatoid factor test in a patient who has only peripheral arthritis should alert you to the possibility of either AS or another of the seronegative spondyloarthropathies. Moreover, arthrocentesis and synovianalysis may also prove useful, since synovial fluid complement values of AS are not depressed as they are in RA[97].

Presence of the HLA-B27 is perhaps the best single laboratory clue. Its absence, however, does not preclude a diagnosis of AS. Moreover, in order to differentiate AS from other causes of back pain, sacroiliac X-ray examination and the HLA-B27 were explored as two screening tests for their relative potential values to the practising clinician[98]. It was concluded that sacroiliac radiography was the discriminator of choice because of greater specificity as well as other practical considerations.

## Roentgenographic findings

The diagnosis of AS must be confirmed by roentgenographic examination[99,100]. With few exceptions[101–103], the earliest changes occur in the sacroiliac joints (Figure 3.6). While it is customary to include frontal and oblique projections initially, additional views, scintigraphy, or other special techniques may be beneficial when preliminary radiographs are normal or equivocal[99,100,104–119]. However, with sup-

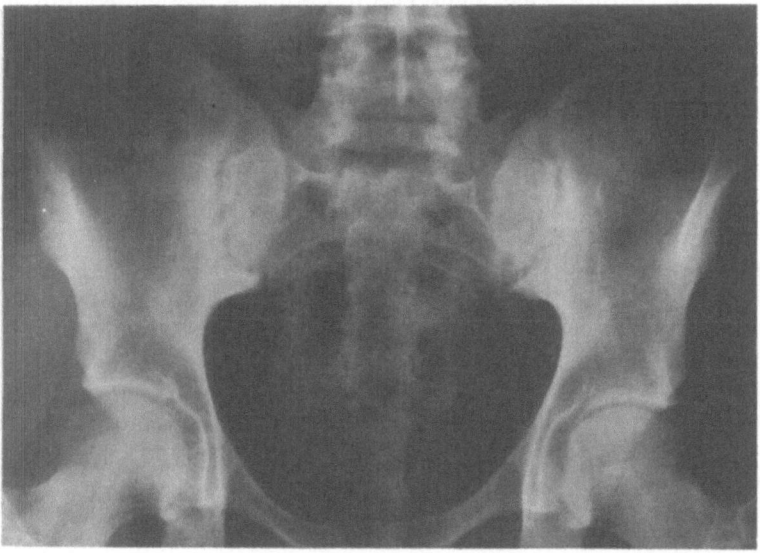

FIGURE 3.6    X-ray of the pelvis discloses pseudowidening of the sacroiliac joints from subchondral erosions and sclerosis that are more prominent on the iliac side

plemental approaches, the skill and experience of the interpreter are
extremely important[99,100,119]. Finally, X-ray abnormalities of the sacroiliac joints are not unique to AS or related spondyloarthropathies and
may occur in a host of other disorders (Table 3.5)[25,120].

Sacroiliac abnormalities by roentgenographic examination may be
disclosed in patients with psoriasis or chronic inflammatory bowel
disease in the absence of sacroiliac, spine, or peripheral joint
complaints. They may also occur in juvenile and adult RA[121–123],
Whipple's disease[124,125], relapsing polychondritis, crystal-induced
synovitis from both gout and pseudogout, osteoarthritis[118], alkap-
tonuria (ochronotic arthropathy), pustulotic arthro-osteitis, and acute
or chronic infections of the sacroiliac joints[120].

X-ray abnormalities of the sacroiliac joints may also be found in
familial Mediterranean fever, hyperparathyroidism, Paget's disease,
Gaucher's disease, osteitis condensans ilii, paraplegia, tuberous sclerosis, fluorosis, occupational acro-osteolysis from vinyl chloride pois-
oning, and traumatic lesions of the sacroiliac joints[120]. The sacroiliac
area is often tender on palpation in fibrositis (fibromyalgia), but the

TABLE 3.5   Disorders associated with roentgenographic abnormalities of the sacroiliac joints

| | |
|---|---|
| Psoriasis* | Hyperparathyroidism |
| Ulcerative colitis* | Paget's disease |
| Regional enteritis* | Gaucher's disease |
| Juvenile rheumatoid arthritis | Osteitis condensans ilii |
| Adult rheumatoid arthritis | Paraplegia |
| Whipple's disease | Tuberous sclerosis |
| Relapsing polychondritis | Fluorosis |
| Gout | Occupational acro-osteolysis from |
| Pseudogout | vinyl chloride poisoning |
| Osteoarthritis | Traumatic lesions of the |
| Ochronotic arthropathy | sacroiliac joint(s) |
| Pustulotic arthro-osteitis | Benign tumours (osteoid osteoma) |
| Acute or chronic infections | Primary and secondary |
| of the sacroiliac joint(s) | malignancies |
| Familial Mediterranean fever | Sacrococcygeal agenesis |

*May be disclosed in these disorders in the absence of sacroiliac, spine, or peripheral joint complaints.

joints are normal on X-ray examination[126]. Benign tumours, including osteoid osteoma[127], as well as both primary and secondary malignancies may also affect the sacroiliac joints. The major congenital anomaly of the joints is sacrococcygeal agenesis[120]. It is frequently combined with anomalies of the lower thoracic and upper lumbar spine.

Early changes of the lumbar spine include diffuse vertebral squaring and demineralization (Figure 3.7). Minimal ligamentous calcification and one or two evolving syndesmophytes may also be noted. The classic 'bamboo spine' with its prominent syndesmophytes and diffuse paraspinal ligamentous calcification (Figure 3.8), the usual textbook illustration, is not useful in early diagnosis. In fact, it takes an average of ten years to develop and evolves only in patients with progressive disease, a group comprising no more than 15% of all patients with AS[128].

## DIFFERENTIAL DIAGNOSIS

The causes of chronic low back pain are so numerous that pinpointing the precise one is often a difficult diagnostic challenge[129-132]. In fact,

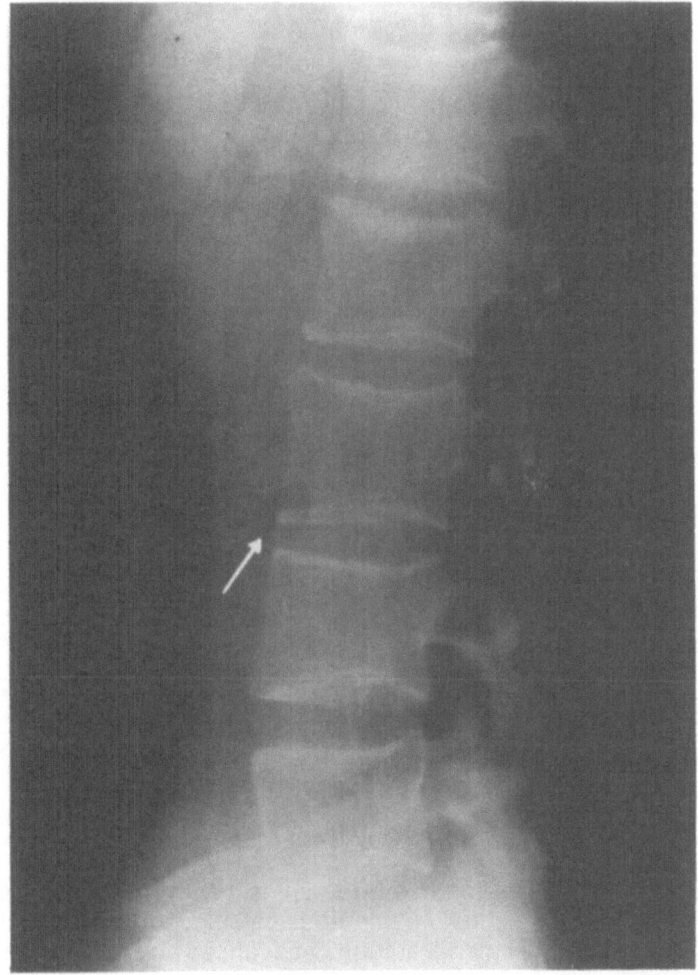

FIGURE 3.7 Lateral X-ray of the lumbar spine reveals typical early changes including demineralization and squaring of vertebral bodies as well as ligamentous calcification from $L_3$ to $L_4$

the physician has to consider a host of possibilities from poor posture to malignancy (Table 3.6)[129].

Herniated intervertebral disk

When only the low back is affected, one of the most important con-

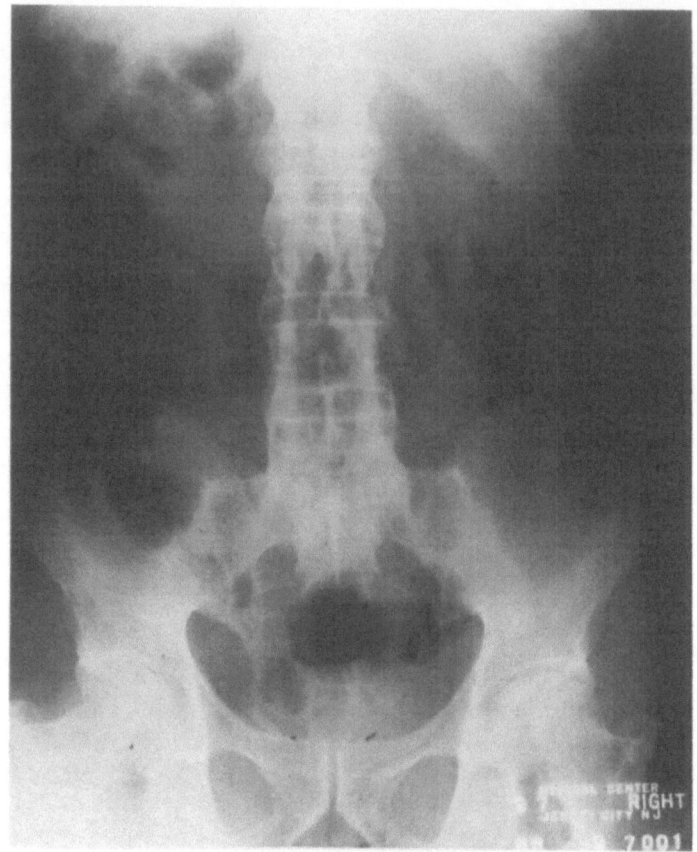

FIGURE 3.8 The classic 'bamboo' spine, with prominent syndes-mophytes, diffuse paraspinal ligamentous calcification, and fused sacro-iliac joints is a late X-ray manifestation of advanced ankylosing spondylitis

ditions to rule out is a herniated lumbar disc. Clearly, this disorder is restricted to the spine, usually begins suddenly rather than insidiously as in AS[130], has no systemic manifestations such as fatigue, anorexia or weight loss, and all laboratory tests, including the ESR, are normal. The only certain way to diagnose a herniated disc is to confirm the defect with either myelography or a CT scan.

Spondylodiscitis, or erosive lesions of the vertebral bodies sur-rounding a disc, has been reported in AS[133-135]. Unlike herniated disc, the spondylodiscitis of AS is frequently asymptomatic and benign,

TABLE 3.6   Causes of chronic low back pain

| Major disorders | Examples |
| --- | --- |
| Structural/functional | Scoliosis/poor posture |
| Pathomechanical | Fracture, dislocation |
| Root compression | Herniated disc, degenerative disc disease |
| Infection | Pott's disease |
| Metabolic | Primary osteoporosis |
| Neoplastic | Multiple myeloma, metastatic malignancy |
| Referred pain | Inflammatory or other chronic disorders of the pelvis or abdomen |
| Rheumatic disorders | Ankylosing spondylitis; Reiter's syndrome, primary fibrositis |

usually evolving late in the course of disease in patients with progressive AS[134,135]. Only rarely is spondylodiscitis a presenting manifestation of AS[135]. There is no agreement on the pathogenesis of this lesion, although trauma with microfractures has been implicated.

## Diffuse idiopathic skeletal hyperostosis

A more difficult differential diagnosis may be offered by the syndrome of diffuse idiopathic skeletal hyperostosis (DISH), also known as Forestier's disease. It occurs primarily in men over the age of 50 and bears a striking resemblance to AS roentgenographically[136]. However, patients with DISH rarely have spinal pain, stiffness, or loss of motion[137]. In DISH, findings on X-ray examination include continuous (flowing) calcification and ossification of the anterolateral aspects of at least three or four contiguous vertebrae that occur most often in the cervical and lower thoracic spine (Figure 3.9). However, the sacroiliac and apophyseal joints, as well as the disc spaces, are not involved in the DISH syndrome. Moreover, the ESR will be normal and the DISH syndrome is not linked to the B27 antigen[138].

## Fibrositis (Fibromyalgia)

Fibrositis, also known as fibromyalgia or fibromyositis, should also be included in the differential diagnosis[126]. It is a common form of non-articular rheumatism characterized by diffuse aches and stiff-

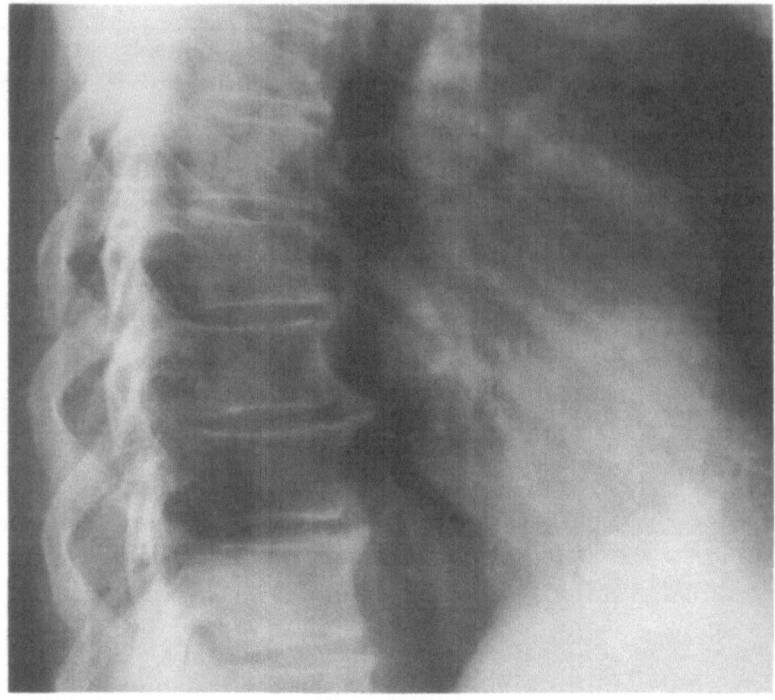

FIGURE 3.9    In diffuse idiopathic skeletal hyperostosis, lateral X-ray of the thoracic spine reveals diffuse (flowing) calcification along the anterior aspect of several contiguous vertebrae. Note that the apophyseal joints and disc spaces are preserved

ness that affects most often young and middle-aged women[126,139]. The syndrome can be primary or secondary to other rheumatic diseases[140].

Patients with fibrositis complain of musculoskeletal pain and stiffness, usually worse in the morning[126]. Common tender sites include the neck, midback, and low back, as well as the elbows, shoulders, anterior chest wall, upper gluteal areas, and knees[141]. The presence of multiple tender points at precisely predictable symmetrical sites confirms the diagnosis[126,142].

As a secondary disorder, fibrositis may occur in patients with AS. In addition to arthritis, the patient now has diffuse aches and pains with typical modulating factors in which symptoms are intensified by cold and damp weather, excessive physical activity, and emotional tension[126]. Consequently, it would be inappropriate to alter the basic drug therapy of AS. Instead, the primary care physician must explain to the patient the basis of these additional complaints. Above all, the benign nature of the fibrositis syndrome should be emphasized. Moreover, regular follow-up care is essential to assume continuous emotional support and other appropriate measures[142–144]. Improvement often follows treatment with tricyclic agents such as low-dose cyclobenzaprine, imipramine, or amytriptyline, by physical measures, or by reduction of stress[142–145].

## Other exclusions

Spinal stenosis occurs primarily in the elderly. Unlike AS, patients usually complain of pain in the back or lower extremities that gets worse when they walk or exercise[131].

Trying to decide whether a patient has psychogenic back pain may be extremely difficult[131]. Nevertheless, patients with no organic basis for back pain will often rate the discomfort as severe and diffuse, varying in intensity throughout the day, and burning hot or throbbing. On the other hand, patients with organic disease usually rate pain as moderate and localized, constant throughout the day, and sharp or aching. It is important to appreciate, however, that the patient with emotional overtones may have underlying organic disease as well.

## WOMEN AND CHILDREN WITH SPONDYLITIS

The onset of AS in women and children is frequently atypical, often beginning with arthritis of peripheral joints and without back complaints. Only months or years later do typical back complaints and other spondylitic manifestations evolve.

## Spondylitis in women

AS is not uncommon in women, as previously believed[132]. Consequently, do not lower your suspicion that AS may be at the root of back or peripheral joint problems just because the patient is a woman. Moreover, AS evolves more slowly in women than in men[146]. Consequently, typical clinical and X-ray features may not evolve for ten or more years[146]. AS also tends to occur later in life in women, often after age 40. In addition, the pattern of spinal involvement on X-ray examination is often different from that found in men[147]. In general, women tend to have: (1) a higher frequency of cervical spine abnormalities; (2) a greater tendency for combined cervical and sacroiliac changes with sparing of the thoracic and lumbar spine; and (3) more frequent and severe osteitis pubis.

Osteitis condensans ilii

AS in women should not be confused with osteitis condensans ilii, a syndrome particularly common in postpartum women that may be related to the strain that delivery imposes on the sacroiliac joints[129]. It is characterized roetgenographically by unilateral or bilateral triangular bony sclerosis of the lower ilium (Figure 3.10). Although low back pain is a common feature of osteitis condensans ilii, patients do not develop limitation of spinal movement, X-ray evidence of spondylitis, or the progressive course seen in AS. Furthermore, as

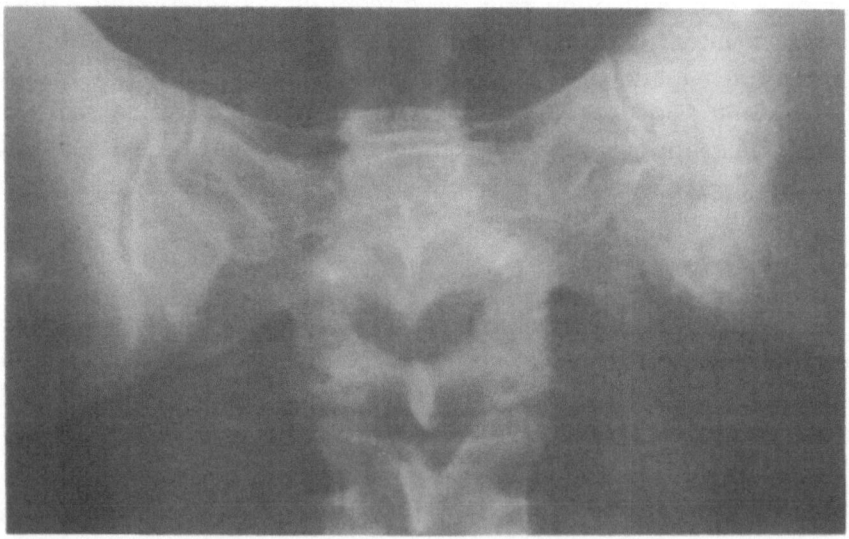

FIGURE 3.10  Sclerosis of the iliac bone is present as triangular or globular densities adjacent to the sacroiliac joints. The sacrum and sacroiliac joints are not involved. Osteitis condensans ilii may affect one or both sides but should not be confused with the sclerosis of ankylosing spondylitis

shown by HLA typing, the frequency of the B27 antigen in osteitis condensans ilii is comparable to that of controls[148]. Consequently, osteitis condensans ilii is not a variant of AS in women, as has been so often suggested in the past.

## Osteoporosis

Primary osteoporosis, which may also be mistaken for AS, is one of the more common causes of backache in the middle-aged and elderly and is particularly prominent in postmenopausal women[129]. Examination often reveals an increased roundness of the back and loss of height, similar to AS. However, unlike AS, back pain is worse when the patient is up and about and is relieved by rest[149]. There are characteristic X-ray changes, including demineralization, wedging, and collapse of vertebrae most frequent in the lower thoracic but also in the lumbar spine.

## Spondylitis in children

Until recently, it has not been appreciated that childhood pauciarthritis (oligoarthritis) may precede and herald the development of spondylitis by years[24,25]. Consequently, AS may be overlooked when the onset occurs in childhood, the condition often being misdiagnosed as pauciarticular juvenile RA[150]. Moreover, while juvenile AS may begin with back complaints it is far more frequent for children to present initially with only peripheral arthritis that may antedate back complaints by 1 to 12 or more years[151-155]. Boys between the ages of 10 and 16 are primarily affected. Additional clues to evolving AS in a child rather than JRA include recurrence of acute (not chronic) anterior uveitis, absence of antinuclear antibodies, and presence of the B27 antigen[152].

An uncommon, yet unique, form of spondylitis, only recently described by Arnett and associates, must also be recognized[156]. Peripheral joint and cervical spine involvement dominate this syndrome that primarily affects girls. The course of disease is characterized by rheumatoid-like hands and limitation of neck motion from cervical apophyseal fusion that progresses into adulthood. In addition to the HLA-B27 antigen, cervical apophyseal fusion is also associated with acute anterior uveitis, micrognathia, sacroiliitis, and spondylitis. Early recognition may be difficult because spondylitic features may be over-shadowed by prominence of peripheral arthritis, especially 'rheu-matoid-like' hand deformities.

## SURVIVAL AND PROGNOSIS

### Survival

Conflicting reports on survival in AS have appeared recently. Of 151 Canadian war veterans observed prospectively since 1947, survival was found to be 61%, significantly less than expected, except for a subgroup of patients not treated with radiotherapy[157]. Another survey disclosed that survivorship of males was no different than that of the general population, while that of females was reduced[158].

### Prognosis

The course and prognosis of AS were examined in two groups, one treated in the 1950s, the other in the 1970s[159]. While the overall prognosis was better in the second group, believed to be the result of general improvement in patient management, there were nevertheless patients with rapidly progressive disease and deformity.

The long-term prognosis is bleakest for patients who develop rapidly progressive arthritis of the spine or hips, for those with underlying ulcerative colitis or regional enteritis, and for the rare patient who develops secondary amyloidosis[160]. Blindness from recurrent anterior uveitis rarely occurs. With early diagnosis, comprehensive manage-ment, and patient compliance, a satisfactory functional capacity can be maintained in most patients who are thus able to lead full and productive lives.

### References

1. Calabro, J. J. (1986). Ankylosing spondylitis: A critical review of current man-agement. *Adv. Ther.*, **3**, 1–20
2. Moll, J. M. H. (1980). *Ankylosing Spondylitis.* (Edinburgh: Churchill Liv-ingstone)
3. Wright, V. and Moll, J. M. H. (1976) *Seronegative Polyarthritis.* (Amsterdam: North Holland)
4. Calin, A. (1984). *Spondylarthropathies.* (Orlando: Grune & Stratton)
5. Calin, A. and Fries, J. F. (1978). *Ankylosing Spondylitis. Discussions in Patient Management.* (Garden City, NY: Medical Examination Publ.)

6. Calabro, J. J. and Kass, E. (1980). Summary of proceedings from a symposium on Bechterew's syndrome. *Scand. J. Rheumatol.*, **9** (Suppl. 32), 247–9
7. Dick, W.C. (1983). Pathogenesis of HLA-B27 associated diseases; summing up. *Br. J. Rheumatol.*, **22** (Suppl. 2), 184–6
8. Calin, A. (1984). Spondylarthropathies: An overview. In Calin, A. (ed.) *Spondylarthropathies*, pp. 1–8. (Orlando: Grune & Stratton)
9. Ott, V. R. (1980). Problems in terminology. *Scand. J. Rheumatol.*, 9 (Suppl. 32), 242
10. Bywaters, E. G. L. (1980). 'Nosonymy and eponymy'. *Scand. J. Rheumatol.*, **9** (Suppl. 32), 242
11. Kass, E. (1980). Syndrome or disease? Use of eponym or symptom-related name? *Scand. J. Rheumatol.*, **9** (Suppl. 32), 240–1
12. Bywaters, E. G. L. (1983). Historical perspectives in the etiology of ankylosing spondylitis. *Br. J. Rheumatol.*, **22** (Suppl. 2), 1–4
13. Calabro, J. J. (1968). An appraisal of the medical and surgical management of ankylosing spondylitis. *Clin. Orthop.*, **60,** 125–48
14. Blumberg, B. S., Bunim, J. J., Calkins, E., Pirani, C. L. and Zvaifler, N. J. (1964). ARA nomenclature and classification of arthritis and rheumatism (tentative). *Arthritis Rheum.*, **7,** 93–7
15. Decker, J. R. (1983). American Rheumatism Association nomenclature and classification of arthritis and rheumatism. *Arthritis Rheum.*, **26,** 1029–32
16. Wright, V., Neuman, V., Shinebaum, R. and Cooke, E. M. (1983). Pathogenesis of seronegative arthritis. *Br. J. Rheumatol.*, **22** (Suppl. 2), 29–32
17. Calabro, J. J. (1980). The spondylarthropathies: An overview. *Scand. J. Rheumatol.*, **9** (Suppl. 32), 21–4
18. Wright, V. (1975). Family studies implicating genetic factors in rheumatic diseases. *Ann. Rheum. Dis.*, **34,** (Suppl. 1), 24–6
19. Wright, V. (1978). Seronegative polyarthritis: A unified concept. *Arthritis Rheum.*, **21,** 619–33
20. Wright, V. (1979). A unifying concept for the spondyloarthropathies. *Clin. Orthop.*, **143,** 8–14
21. Moll, J. M. H. (1983). Pathogenetic mechanisms in B27 associated diseases. *Br. J. Rheumatol.*, **22** (Suppl. 2), 93–103
22. Ball, J. (1983). The enthesopathy of ankylosing spondylitis. *Br. J. Rheumatol.*, **22** (Suppl. 2), 25–8
23. Calabro, J. J. (1986). The seronegative spondyloarthopathies. A graduated approach to management. *Postgrad. Med.*, **80,** 173–88
24. Calabro, J. J. (1983). Clinical aspects of juvenile and adult ankylosing spondylitis. *Br. J. Rheumatol.*, **22** (Suppl. 2), 104–9
25. Calabro, J. J. (1985). Drug therapy of juvenile rheumatoid arthritis and the seronegative spondyloarthropathies. In Roth, S. H. (ed.) *Handbook of Drug Therapy in Rheumatology*, pp. 115–80. (Littleton, MA: PSG Publ. Co.)
26. Moll, J. H. M., Haslock, I., Macrae, I. F. and Wright, V. (1974). Associations between ankylosing spondylitis, psoriatic arthritis, Reiter's disease, the intestinal arthropathies and Behçet's syndrome. *Medicine*, **53,** 343–64
27. Wright, V. (1980). Relationships between ankylosing spondylitis and other spondarthritides. In Moll, J. M. H. (ed.). *Ankylosing Spondylitis*. pp. 42–51. (Edinburgh: Churchill Livingstone)
28. Brewerton, D. A., Caffrey, M., Hart, F. D., James, D. C. O., Nicholls, A. and Sturrock, R. D. (1973). Ankylosing spondylitis and HL-A 27. *Lancet*, **1,** 904–7

71

29. Schlosstein, L., Terasaki, P. I., Bluestone, R. and Pearson, C.M. (1973). High association of the HL-A antigen, W27, with ankylosing spondylitis. *N. Engl. J. Med.*, **288**, 704–6
30. Strosberg, J. M., Allen, F. H., Calabro, J. J. and Harris, E. D., Jr (1975). Ankylosing spondylitis in a large kindred: Clinical and genetic studies. *Tissue Antigens*, **5**, 205–12
31. Kass, E. and Vinje, O. (1983). Pathogenesis of ankylosing spondylitis and related disorders: Future perspectives. *Br. J. Rheumatol.*, **22** (Suppl. 2), 177–83
32. Carter, M. E. (1980). Epidemiology. In Moll, J. M. H. (ed.) *Ankylosing Spondylitis*, pp. 16–25. (Edinburgh: Churchill Livingstone)
33. Woodrow, J. C. (1980). Genetics. In Moll. J. M. H. (ed.)*Ankylosing Spondylitis*, pp. 26–41. (Edinburgh: Churchill Livingstone)
34. Bywaters, E. G. L. (1980). Historical introduction. In Moll, J. M. H. (ed.) *Ankylosing Spondylitis*, pp. 1–15. (Edinburgh: Churchill Livingstone)
35. Ebringer, R. W., Cawdell, D. R., Cowling P. and Ebringer, A. (1978). Sequential studies in ankylosing spondylitis; association of *Klebsiella pneumoniae* with active disease. *Ann. Rheum. Dis.*, **37**, 146–51
36. Ebringer, A., Baines, M., Childerstone, M., Ghuloom, M. and Ptaszynska T. (1985). Etiopathogenesis of ankylosing spondylitis and the cross-tolerance hypothesis. In Ziff, M. and Cohen, S. B. (eds.) *The Spondyloarthropathies*, pp. 101–28. (New York: Raven Press)
37. van Bohemen Ch, H. G., Nabbe, A. J. J. M., Goei The H. S., Dekker-Saeys, A. J. and Zanen, H. C. (1986). Antibodies to enterobacteriaceae in ankylosing spondylitis. *Scand. J. Rheumatol.*, **15**, 143–7
38. Calin, A. and Fries, J. F. (1975). The striking prevalence of ankylosing spondylitis in 'healthy' W27 positive males and females. A controlled study. *N. Engl. J. Med.*, **293**, 835–9
39. Khan, M. A. (1984) Spondylarthritis in non-Caucasians. In Calin, A. (ed.) *Spondylarthropathies*, pp. 265–77. (New York: Grune & Stratton)
40. Arnett, F. C. (1984). HLA and the spondylarthropathies. In Calin, A. (ed.) *Spondylarthropathies*, pp. 297–321. (New York: Grune & Stratton)
41. Calin, A., Fries, J. F., Schurman, D. and Payne, R. (1977). The close correlation between symptoms and disease expression in HLA-B27 positive individuals. *J. Rheumatol.*, **4**, 277–81
42. Cohen, L. M., Mittal, K. K., Schmid, F. R., Rogers, L. F. and Cohen, K. L. (1976). Increased risk for spondylitis stigmata in apparently healthy HL-A W27 men. *Ann. Intern. Med.*, **84**, 1–7
43. Rothova, A., Buitenhuis, H. J., Christiaana, B. J., Linssen, A., van der Gaag, R., Kijlstra, A. and Feltkamp, T. E. W. (1983). Acute anterior uveitis (AAU) and HLA-B27. *Br. J. Rheumatol.*, **22** (Suppl. 2), 144–5
44. van der Linden, S., Valkenburg, H. A. and Cats, A. (1983). Is uveitis associated with ankylosing spondylitis or with HLA-B27? *Br. J. Rheumatol.*, **22** (Suppl. 2), 146–7
45. White, L. F., McCoy, R. J., Tait, B. and Ebringer, R. (1983). Acute anterior uveitis: A model for HLA-B27 associated diseases. *Br. J. Rheumatol.*, **22** (Suppl. 2), 148–50
46. Maltz, B. A., Sussman, P. and Calabro, J. J. (1969). Peripheral arthritis as an initial manifestation of ankylosing spondylitis. *Arthritis Rheum.*, **12**, 680–1

47. Calabro, J. J., Londino, A. V., Jr and Eyvazzadeh, C. (1985). Ankylosing spondylitis: Clues to early diagnosis: Part I. *Clin. Rheumatol. Prac.*, **3**, 143–54
48. Polley, H. F. and Slocumb, C. H. (1947). Rheumatoid spondylitis: A study of 1,035 cases. *Ann. Intern. Med.*, **26**, 240–9
49. Russell, A. S., Lentle, B. C., Percy, J. S. and Jackson, F. I. (1975). Scintigraphy of sacroiliac joints in acute anterior uveitis. *Ann. Intern. Med.*, **85**, 606–8
50. Kinsella, P., Ebringer, R., Hooker, J., Corbett, M., Cox, N. and Wynn Parry, C. B. (1978). Ankylosing spondylitis presenting as PUO. *Br. Med. J.*, **1**, 19–20
51. Resnick, D. (1974). Patterns of peripheral joint disease in ankylosing spondylitis. *Radiology*, **110**, 523–32
52. Dwosh, I. L., Resnick D. and Becker, M. A. (1976). Hip involvement in ankylosing spondylitis. *Arthritis Rheum.*, **19**, 683–92
53. Marks, J. S. and Hardinge, K. (1979). Clinical and radiographic features of ankylosing spondylitis hip disease. *Ann. Rheum. Dis.*, **38**, 332–6
54. Scott, D. L., Eastmond, C. J. and Wright, V. (1979). A comparative radiological study of the pubic symphysis in rheumatic disorders. *Ann. Rheum. Dis.*, **38**, 529–34
55. Reuler, J. B., Girard, D. E. and Nardone, D. A. (1978). Sternoclavicular joint involvement in ankylosing spondylitis. *South Med. J.*, **71**, 1480–1
56. Davidson, C., Wojtulewski, J. A., Bacon, P. A. and Winstock, D. (1975). Temporo-mandibular joint disease in ankylosing spondylitis *Ann. Rheum. Dis.*, **34**, 87–9
57. Resnick, D. (1974). Temporomandibular joint involvement in ankylosing spondylitis. *Radiology*, **112**, 29–35
58. Berendes, J. and Miehlke, A. (1973). A rare ankylosis of the cricoarytenoid joints. *Arch. Otolaryngol.*, **98**, 63–5
59. Wojtulewski, J. A., Sturrock, R. D., Branfoot, A. C. and Hart, F. D. (1973). Cricoarytenoid arthritis in ankylosing spondylitis. *Br. Med. J.*, **3**, 145–6
60. Resnick, D., Feingold, M. I., Curd, J., Niwayama G. and Goergen, T. G. (1977). Calcaneal abnormalities in articular disorders: rheumatoid arthritis, ankylosing spondylitis, psoriatic arthritis, and Reiter's syndrome. *Radiology*, **125**, 355–66
61. Gerster, J. C., Vischer, T. L., Bennani, A. and Fallet, G. H. (1977). The painful heel. Comparative study in rheumatoid arthritis, ankylosing spondylitis, Reiter's syndrome, and generalized osteoarthrosis. *Ann. Rheum. Dis.*, **36**, 343–8
62. Gerster, J. C., Hauser, H. and Fallet, G. H. (1975). Xeroradiographic techniques applied to assessment of Achilles tendon in inflammatory or metabolic diseases. *Ann. Rheum. Dis.*, **34**, 479–88
63. Enright, T., Liang, G. C., Fox, T. A. and Mueller R. F. (1979). Tarsal tunnel syndrome with ankylosing spondylitis. *Arthritis Rheum.*, **22**, 77–9
64. Khan, M. A., Kushner, I. and Braun, W. E. (1977). Comparison of clinical features in HLA-27 positive and negative patients with ankylosing spondylitis. *Arthritis Rheum.*, **20**, 909–11
65. Hart, F. D. (1980). Clinical features and complications. In Moll, J. M. H. (ed.) *Ankylosing Spondylitis*, pp. 52–68. (Edinburgh: Churchill Livingstone)
66. Forouzesh, S. and Bluestone, R. (1979). The clinical spectrum of ankylosing spondylitis. *Clin. Orthop.*, **143**, 53–8
67. Cumming, W. J. K. and Saunders, M. (1978). Radiculopathy as a complication of ankylosing spondylitis. *J. Neurol. Neurosurg. Psychiatry*, **41**, 569–70
68. Thomas, D. J., Kendall, M. J. and Whitfield, A. G. W. (1974). Nervous system involvement in ankylosing spondylitis. *Br. Med. J.*, **1**, 148–50

73

69. Osgood, C., Martin, L. G. and Ackerman, E. (1973). Fracture-dislocation of the cervical spine with ankylosing spondylitis. *J. Neurosurg.*, **39**, 764–9
70. Davidson, R. I. and Tyler, H. R. (1974). Bulbar symptoms and episodic aphonia associated with atlanto-occipital subluxation in ankylosing spondylitis. *J. Neurol. Neurosurg. Psychiatry*, **37**, 691–5
71. Little, H., Swinson, D. R. and Cruickshank, B. (1976). Upward subluxation of the Axis in ankylosing spondylitis. A clinical pathologic report. *Am. J. Med.*, **60**, 279–85
72. Hassan, I. (1976). Cauda equina syndrome in ankylosing spondylitis: A report of six cases. *J. Neurol. Neurosurg. Psychiatry*, **39**, 1172–8
73. Russell, M. L., Gordon, D. A., Ogryzlo, M. A. and McPhedran, R. S. (1973). The cauda equina syndrome of ankylosing spondylitis. *Ann. Intern. Med.*, **78**, 551–4
74. Gordon, A. L. and Yudell, A. (1973). Cauda equina lesion associated with rheumatoid spondylitis. *Ann. Intern. Med.*, **78**, 555–7
75. Gordon, D. A., Russell, M. L., Ogryzlo, M. A. and McPhedran, R. S. (1973). Ankylosing spondylitis (letter). *Ann. Intern. Med.*, **79**, 139–40
76. Weed, C. L., Kulander, B. G., Mazzarella, J. A. and Decker, J. L. (1966). Heart block in ankylosing spondylitis. *Arch. Intern. Med.*, **35**, 145–62
77. Kinsella, T. D., Johnson, L. G. and Sutherland, R. I. (1974). Cardiovascular manifestations of ankylosing spondylitis. *Can. Med. Assoc. J.*, **111**, 1309–11
78. Bulkley, B. H. and Roberts, W. C. (1973). Ankylosing spondylitis and aortic regurgitation. *Circulation*, **48**, 1014–27
79. Roberts, W. C., Hollingsworth, J. F., Bulkley, B. H., Jaffe, R. B., Epstein, S. E. and Stinson, E. B. (1974). Combined and aortic regurgitation in ankylosing spondylitis. *Am. J. Med.*, **56**, 237–43
80. Spitzer, S., Peguero, F. and Mason, D. (1975). Rheumatoid spondylitis, aortic insufficiency and coronary artery disease. *Chest*, **68**, 828–9
81. Harvey, D. B., Hollenberg, M., Kunkel, F. and Scheinman, M. M. (1976). Ankylosing spondylitis with complete heart block. *Arch. Intern. Med.*, **136**, 1046–50
82. Alexander, B. and Feiner, H. (1979). Ankylosing spondylitis with cardiac dysrhythmia. *NY State J. Med.*, **79**, 1585–8
83. Hart, F. D., Emerson, P. A. and Gregg, I. (1963). Thorax in ankylosing spondylitis. *Ann. Rheum. Dis.*, **22**, 11–18
84. Citrin, D. L., Boyd, G. and Bradley, G. W. (1973). Ventilatory function and transfer factor in ankylosing spondylitis *Scott. Med. J.*, **18**, 109–13
85. Rosenow III, E. C., Strimlan, C. V., Muhm, J. R. and Ferguson, R. H. (1977). Pleuropulmonary manifestations of ankylosing spondylitis. *Mayo Clin. Proc.*, **52**, 641–9
86. Appelrouth, D. and Gottlieb, N. L. (1975). Pulmonary manifestations of ankylosing spondylitis. *J. Rheumatol.*, **2**, 446–53
87. Wolson, A. H. and Rohwedder, J. J. (1975). Upper lobe fibrosis in ankylosing spondylitis. *Am. J. Roentgenol. Radium Ther. Nucl. Med.*, **124**, 466–71
88. Gupta, S. M. and Johnston, W. H. (1978). Apical pulmonary disease in ankylosing spondylitis. *NZ Med. J.*, **88**, 186–8
89. Stiksa, G., Eklundh, G., Riebe, I. and Simonsson, B. G. (1976). Bilateral pulmonary aspergilloma in ankylosing spondylitis treated with transthoracic intracavitary instillations of antifungal agents. *Scand. J. Respir. Dis.*, **57**, 163–70

90. Calin, A., Porta, J., Fries, J. F. and Schurman, D. J. (1977). Clinical history as a screening test for ankylosing spondylitis. *J. Am. Med. Assoc.*, **237**, 2613–14
91. Laine, V. A. (1980). Non-immunological laboratory findings in Bechterew's syndrome and allied disorders. Diagnostic value and relation to etiology and pathogenesis. *Scand. J. Rheumatol.*, **9** (Suppl. 32), 47–9
92. Sturrock, R. D. (1980). Laboratory features. In Moll, J. M. H. (ed.) *Ankylosing Spondylitis*, pp. 113–19. (Edinburgh: Churchill Livingstone)
93. Calin, A. (1975). Raised serum creatine phosphokinase activity in ankylosing spondylitis. *Ann. Rheum. Dis.*, **34**, 244–8
94. Kendall, M. J., Lawrence, D. S., Shuttleworth, G. R. and Whitfield, A. G. W. (1973). Rheumatology and biochemistry of ankylosing spondylitis. *Br. Med. J.*, **2**, 235–7
95. Ludwig, A. O., Short, C. L. and Bauer, W. (1943). Rheumatoid arthritis as a cause of increased cerebro-spinal fluid protein; a study of one hundred and one patients. *N. Engl. J. Med.*, **228**, 306–10
96. Calabro, J. J. and Mody R. E. (1966). Management of ankylosing spondylitis. *Bull. Rheum. Dis.*, **16**, 408–11
97. Calabro, J. J., Katz, R. M. and Maltz, B. A. (1969). Ankylosing spondylitis (letter). *J. Pediatr.*, **75**, 912–13
98. Grahame, R., Kennedy, L. and Wood, P. H. N. (1975). HL-A27 and the diagnosis of back problems. *Rheumatol. Rehabil.*, **14**, 168–72
99. Percy, J. S. and Lentle, B. (1980). Radiological and scintigraphic features. In Moll, J. M. H. (ed). *Ankylosing Spondylitis*, pp. 76–86. (Edinburgh: Churchill Livingstone)
100. Greenway, G. D. and Resnick, D. (1980). Problems in radiographic technique and in radiological assessment of the sacroiliac joints. In Moll, J. M. H. (ed.) *Ankylosing Spondylitis*, pp. 87–95. (Edinburgh: Churchill Livingstone)
101. Calin, A. (1979). Ankylosing spondylitis sine sacroilitis. *Arthritis Rheum.*, **22**, 303–4
102. Courtois, C., Fallet, G. H., Visher, T. L. and Wettstein, P. (1980). Erosive spondylopathy. *Ann. Rheum. Dis.*, **39**, 462–9
103. Goei The, H. S. and Cats, A. (1986). Follow-up findings in three patients with spinal ankylosing spondylitis. *Scand. J. Rheumatol.*, **15**, 221–3
104. Chalmers, I. M., Lentle, B. C., Percy, J. S. and Russell, A. S. (1979). Sacroiliitis detected by bone scintiscanning: a clinical, radiological, and scintigraphic follow-up study. *Ann. Rheum. Dis.*, **38**, 112–17
105. Domeij-Nyberg, B., Kjallman, M., Nylen, O. and Pettersson, N. (1980). The reliability of quantitative bone scanning in sacro-iliitis. *Scand. J. Rheumatol.*, **9**, 77–9
106. Dunn, E. C., Ebringer, R. W. and Ell, P. J. (1980). Quantitative scintigraphy in the early diagnosis of sacro-iliitis. *Rheumatol. Rehab.*, **19**, 69–75
107. Esdaile, J., Hawkins, D. and Rosenthall, L. (1979). Radionuclide joint imaging in the seronegative spondyloarthropathies. *Clin. Orthop.*, **143**, 46–52
108. Ho, G. Jr, Sadovnikoff, N., Malhotra, C. M. and Claunch, B. C. (1979). Quantitative sacroiliac joint scintigraphy: A critical assessment. *Arthritis Rheum.*, **22**, 837–44
109. Spencer, D. G., Adams, F. G., Horton, P. W. and Buchanan, W. W. (1979). Scintiscanning in ankylosing spondylitis: A clinical, radiological and quantitative radioisotopic study. *J. Rheumatol.*, **6**, 426–31

110. Esdaile, J. M., Rosenthall, L., Terkeltaud, R. and Kloiber, R. (1980). Prospective evaluation of sacroiliac scintigraphy in chronic inflammatory back pain. *Arthritis Rheum.*, **23**, 998–1003
111. Szanto, E. and Ruden, B. (1976). $^{99m}$Tc in evaluation of sacro-iliac arthritis. *Scand. J. Rheumatol.*, **5**, 11–15
112. Russell, A. S., Lentle, B. C. and Percy, J. S. (1975). Investigation of sacroiliac disease: Comparative evaluation of radiological and radionuclide techniques. *J. Rheumatol.*, **2**, 45–51
113. Russell, A. S., Lentle, B. C. and Schlaut, J. (1976). Radiologic and scintiscan findings in HLA-B27 negative patients with ankylosing spondylitis. *J. Rheumatol.*, **3**, 321–3
114. Berghs, H., Remans, J., Drieskens, L., Kiebooms, L. and Polderman, J. (1978). Diagnostic value of sacroiliac joint scintigraphy with $^{99m}$technetium pyrophosphate in sacroiliitis. *Ann. Rheum. Dis.*, **37**, 190–4
115. Szanto, E. and Lindvall, N. (1978). Quantitative $^{99m}$Tc pertechnetate scanning of the sacroiliac joints. A follow-up study of patients with suspected sacro-iliitis. *Scand. J. Rheumatol.*, **7**, 93–6
116. Namey, T. C., McIntyre, Jr, Buse, M. and LeRoy, E. C. (1977). Nucleographic studies of axial spondarthritides. I. Quantitative sacroiliac scintigraphy in early HLA-B27-associated sacroiliitis. *Arthritis Rheum.*, **20**, 1058–64
117. Dory, M. A. and Francois, R. J. (1978) Craniocaudal axial view of the sacroiliac joint. *Am. J. Roentgenol.*, **130**, 1125–31
118. Resnick, D., Niwayama, G. and Goergen, T. G. (1977). Comparison of radiographic abnormalities of the sacroiliac joint in degenerative disease and ankylosing spondylitis. *Am. J. Roentgenol.*, **128**, 189–96
119. Goldberg, R. P., Genant, H. K., Shimshak, R. and Shames, D. (1978). Applications and limitations of quantitative sacroiliac joint scintigraphy. *Radiology*, **128**, 683–6
120. Bellamy, N., Park, W. and Rooney, P. J. (1983). What do we know about the sacroiliac joint? *Semin. Arthritis Rheum.*, **12**, 282–313
121. Dahlqvist, S. R., Nordmark, L. G. and Bjelle, A. (1984). HLA-B27 and involvement of sacroiliac joints in rheumatoid arthritis. *J. Rheumatol.*, **11**, 27–32
122. Sharp, J. T. O. Calkins, E., Cohen, A. S., Schubart, A. F. and Calabro, J. J. (1964). Observations on the clinical, chemical, and serological manifestations of rheumatoid arthritis, based on the course of 154 cases. *Medicine*, **43**, 41–58
123. Carter, M. E. (1962). Sacro-iliitis in Still's disease. *Ann. Rheum. Dis.*, **21**, 105–20
124. Khan, M. A. (1982). Axial arthropathy in Whipple's disease. *J. Rheumatol.*, **9**, 928–9
125. Conoso, J. J., Saini, M. and Hermos, J. (1978). Whipple's disease and ankylosing spondylitis; simultaneous occurrence in HLA-B27 positive male. *J. Rheumatol.*, **5**, 79–84
126. Yunus, M., Masi, A. T., Calabro, J. J., Miller, K. A. and Fergenbaum, S. L. (1981). Primary fibromyalgia (fibrositis): Clinical study of 50 patients with matched normal controls. *Semin. Arthritis Rheum.*, **11**, 151–71
127. Cohen, M. D., Harrington, T. M. and Ginsburg, W. W. (1983). Osteoid osteoma: 95 cases and a review of the literature. *Semin. Arthritis Rheum.*, **12**, 265–81
128. Gran, J. T., Husby, G., Hordvik, M., Stormer, J. and Romberg-Andersen, O. (1984). Radiological changes in men and women with ankylosing spondylitis. *Ann. Rheum. Dis.*, **43**, 570–5.

129. Calabro, J. J. (1982). Diagnosis of low back pain. In Stanton-Hicks, M. and Boas, R. (eds.) *Chronic Low Back Pain*, pp. 39–57. (New York: Raven Press)
130. Dixon, A. St J. and Macleod, M. (1980). Diagnostic problems and differential diagnosis. In Moll, J. M. H. (ed.) *Ankylosing Spondylitis*, pp. 151–62. (Edinburgh: Churchill Livingstone)
131. Hockberger, R. (1986). The lowdown on low back pain. *Emergency Med.*, **18**, 122–71
132. Arnett, F. C., Khan, M. A. and Willkens, R. F. (1986). Backache: Are you missing ankylosing spondylitis? *Patient Care*, **20**, 51–78
133. Modena, V., Migone, N., Daneo, V., Carbonara, O., di Vittorio, S. and Viara, M. (1978). Spondylodiscitis and ankylosing spondylitis: HLA typing and nosological implications. *Ann. Rheum. Dis.*, **37**, 510–12
134. Little, H., Urowitz, M. B., Smythe, H. A. and Rosen, P. S. (1974). Asymptomatic spondylodiscitis. An unusual feature of ankylosing spondylitis. *Arthritis Rheum.*, **17**, 487–93
135. Bourqui, M. and Gerster, J. C. (1985). Ankylosing spondylitis presenting as spondylodiscitis. *Clin. Rheumatol.*, **4**, 458–64
136. Resnick, D., Shapiro, R. F., Wiesner, K. B., Newayama, G., Utsinger, P. D. and Shaul, S. R. (1978). Diffuse idiopathic skeletal hyperostosis (DISH) (ankylosing hyperostosis of Forestier and Rotes-Querol). *Semin. Arthritis Rheum.*, **7**, 153–87
137. Rothschild, B. M. (1985). Diffuse idiopathic skeletal hyperostosis: Misconceptions and reality. *Clin. Rheum. Prac.*, **3**, 207–12
138. Ercilla, M. G., Brancos, M. A., Breysse, G. A., Alonso, G., Vives, J., Castillo, R. and Querol, J. R. (1977). HLA antigens in Forestier's disease, ankylosing spondylitis, and polyarthrosis of the hands. *J. Rheumatol.*, **4** (Suppl. 3), 89–93
139. Smythe, H. A. and Moldofsky, H. (1977). Two contributions to understanding of the 'fibrositis' syndrome. *Bull. Rheum. Dis.*, **28**, 928–31
140. Wolfe, F. and Cathey, M. A. (1983). Prevalence of primary and secondary fibrositis. *J. Rheumatol.*, **10**, 965–8
141. Smythe, H. (1986). Tender points: Evolution of concepts of the fibrositis/fibromyalgia syndrome. *Am. J. Med.*, **81** (Suppl. 3A), 2–6
142. Wolfe, F. (1986). The clinical syndrome of fibrositis. *Am. J. Med.*, **81** (Suppl. 3A), 7–14
143. Bennett, R. M. (1986). Current issues concerning the management of the fibrositis/fibromyalgia syndrome. *Am. J. Med.*, **81** (Suppl. 3A), 15–18
144. Gatter, R. A. (1986). Pharmacotherapeutics in fibrositis. *Am. J. Med.*, **81** (Suppl. 3A), 63–6
145. Hench, P. K. (1986). Secondary fibrositis. *Am. J. Med.*, **81** (Suppl. 3A), 60–2
146. Hill, H. F. H., Hill, A. G. S. and Bodmer, J. G. (1976). Clinical diagnosis of ankylosing spondylitis in women and relation to presence of HLA-B27. *Ann. Rheum. Dis.*, **35**, 267–70
147. Resnick, D., Dowsh, I. L., Goergen, T. G., Shapiro, R. F., Utsinger, P. D., Wiesner, K. B. and Bryan, D. L. (1976). Clinical and radiographic abnormalities in ankylosing spondylitis – comparison of men and women. *Radiology*, **119**, 293–7
148. Singal, D. P., de Bosset, P., Gordon, D. A., Smythe, H. A., Urowitz, M. B. and Koehler, B. E. (1977). HLA antigens in osteitis condensans and ankylosing spondylitis. *J. Rheumatol.*, **4** (Suppl. 3), 105–8

149. Sarkin, T. L. (1977). Backache in the aged. *S. Afr. Med. J.*, **51,** 418–20
150. Calabro, J. J., Holgerson, W. B., Sonpal, G. B. and Khoury, M. I. (1976). Juvenile rheumatoid arthritis. A general review and report of 100 patients observed for 15 years. *Semin. Arthritis Rheum.*, **5,** 257–98
151. Bywaters, E. G. L. (1976). Ankylosing spondylitis in childhood. *Clin. Rheum. Dis.*, **87,** 387–96
152. Calabro, J. J., Gordon, R. D. and Miller, K. A. (1980). Bechterew's syndrome in children: Diagnostic criteria. *Scand. J. Rheumatol.*, **9** (Suppl. 32), 45–6
153. Marks, S., Barnett, M. and Calin, A. (1981). The natural history of juvenile ankylosing spondylitis: A case controlled study of juvenile and adult onset disease (Abst). *Arthritis Rheum.*, **24,** S79
154. Rosenberg, A. M. and Petty, R. E. (1982). A syndrome of seronegative enthesopathy and arthropathy in children. *Arthritis Rheum.*, **25,** 1041–7
155. Schaller, J. G. (1977). Ankylosing spondylitis. *Arthritis Rheum.*, **20** (Suppl.), 398–401
156. Arnett, F. C., Bias, W. B. and Stevens, M. B. (1980). Juvenile-onset chronic arthritis: Clinical and roentgenographic features of a unique HLA-B27 subset. *Am. J. Med.*, **69,** 369–76
157. Kaprove, R. E., Little, A. H., Graham, D. C. and Rosen, P. S. (1980). Ankylosing spondylitis: Survival in men with and without radiotherapy. *Arthritis Rheum.*, **23,** 57–61
158. Carter, E. T., McKenna, C. H., Brian, D. D. and Kurland, L. T. (1979). Epidemiology of ankylosing spondylitis in Rochester, Minnesota, 1935–1973. *Arthritis Rheum.*, **22,** 365–70
159. Lehtinen, K. (1979). Clinical and radiological features of ankylosing spondylitis in the 1950's and 1976 at the same hospital. *Scand. J. Rheumatol.*, **8,** 57–61
160. Husby, G. (1980). Amyloidosis in ankylosing spondylitis. *Scand. J. Rheumatol.*, **9** (Suppl. 32), 57–61

# 4

# ANKYLOSING SPONDYLITIS:
## Clinical Aspects, Comparisons, Men versus Women, Hospitalized versus Epidemiological Patients

*G. HUSBY and J. T. GRAN*

Ankylosing spondylopathies have occurred among animals and man since pre-historic time[1]. The Greek author Pausanias described about year 100 AD[2] the corpse of an Olympic winner, Protophanes, 'which had ribs not separated but joined together from shoulders to the smallest ribs', and this may represent the very first description of ankylosing spondylitis (AS). However, the Irish physician Bernhard Connor was in 1693 the first to describe a condition which was undoubtedly ankylosing spondylitis[3]. Strümpell, Marie, and particularly von Bechterew have got their names linked to AS through their descriptions of this rheumatic disorder in the late nineteenth century[1].

A variety of names have been used for AS: among them the terms pelvospondylitis ossificans (Sweden), Marie–Strümpell's disease (French-speaking countries), and Bechterew's disease or syndrome[4] (Europe) are still used.

Symmetric sacroiliitis is the cardinal feature of ankylosing spondylitis. A useful *working definition* for AS may therefore be symptomatic bilateral sacroiliitis, although its clinical picture may vary from simple sacroiliitis to a severe, progressive systemic disorder[5]. This implies that radiological sacroiliitis which never causes symptoms is not included in this practical definition of AS.

The aetiology of AS is not clear, but it is thought to be multi-factorial[6]. The discovery of the close association between the tissue antigen HLA-B27 and AS (described in detail in another chapter of this volume) clearly demonstrated the importance of genetic factors[7,8], and thus supported previous studies[9-12] reporting a significant familial aggregation of this disease. Environmental factors are apparently also involved[13,14], and triggering factors may be microbial constituents or products[15,16].

The prevalence of AS shows geographic (ethnic) variations related to the frequency of HLA-B27 in the population, but has generally thought to be less than 0.2%. After the introduction of HLA typing the prevalence was found by some workers[17] to be about 10-fold this estimate, i.e. approximately 2%, and the apparent dominance of AS among men was no longer so obvious. Other surveys employing typing for HLA-B27[18] have, however, not revealed a higher prevalence of AS which was still found to be 0.1% or less. In our recent population survey of AS in Tromsø, Northern Norway[19], the prevalence of AS was found to be 1.1–1.4% in a population with a frequency of HLA-B27 of approximately 16%. We believe that the relatively high prevalence of the disease may reflect the similarly increased frequency of the predisposing tissue antigen HLA-B27 in this population. Clearly, the occurrence of AS, and also the prevalence of this disorder among HLA-B27-positive persons are matters of controversy.

The pathology of AS is characterized by enchondral ossification of discs and joint capsules, sometimes leading to bony ankylosis, preceded by a stage of erosive inflammation, and osteolytic destruction of parts of the axial skeleton[20]. The lesions of ankylosing spondylitis are mainly localized to the sacroiliac joints, the intervertebral discs and apophyseal joints of the spine and proximal joints of the extremities[21]. Another characteristic manifestation is the enthesopathy (see elsewhere, this volume) which is an inflammatory erosive lesion localized to attachments of ligaments and tendons leading to apposition of new bone and spur formation[22]. The enthesis is considered to be a fundamental lesion in AS which, however, is a systemic chronic inflammatory disorder that may affect many organs.

# CLINICAL FEATURES OF ANKYLOSING SPONDYLITIS

## Symptoms

The average age at onset of AS is between 24–26 years[23,24], and reportedly up to 70% of the patients experience their initial complaints at an age between 20 and 40 years[9,25]. Onset of symptoms after 40 years occurs in less than 16% of the patients [9,26,27]. Some of the patients are able to relate the disease onset to special events such as trauma, exposure to excessive fatigue, shock, or infection[24,27]. In the majority of the cases, however, the onset is insidious[24,25,27–29], but an acute onset of symptoms is noted in many patients, reportedly between 20 and 57%[25,27,29]. Up to 90% of the patients report low back or lumbar pain as their first symptom[24–26,30]. Other initial sites may be the thoracic spine[15,26,31,32], neck and shoulders[24,26,31], hips[26,27] and peripheral joints[24,26,31]. In one study[31] a monoarticular affection of the knee was the initial symptom in 11% of the patients. The tendon attachments are initially affected in 10–40% of patients, and the pain is often referred to the back of the heels, the ischial tuberosities and the major trochanters[33]. Other manifestations, e.g. acute anterior uveitis, may also sometimes precede the spinal symptoms of AS.

The clinical features reflect the chronic inflammatory nature of AS, which is considered to be the prototype of the seronegative spondylarthropathies, which also include Reiter's syndrome, the psoriatic and the enteric arthropathies, cases of juvenile rheumatoid arthritis and possibly Behcet's syndrome[34]. These disorders have *common associations* which include negative tests for rheumatoid factors, absence of rheumatic nodules, radiological sacroiliitis with or without spondylitis, peripheral arthritis particularly of large, weight-bearing joints, mucocutaneous, genital or gastrointestinal manifestations, tendency to cluster in families and high prevalence of HLA-B27[34]. The inflammatory and ankylosing processes result in pain, tenderness, stiffness (Figure 4.1) and occasionally kyphosis of the spine, decreasing chest expansion, arthritis of larger, peripheral joints, and symptoms from attachments of ligaments and tendons, particularly in the heels, pelvis and chest.

*Back pain* is the cardinal symptom of AS. The pain which is due to *sacroiliitis* is often referred by the patients to the buttocks or hips. The *spondylitic* pain most often starts in the lumbar or dorsolumbar

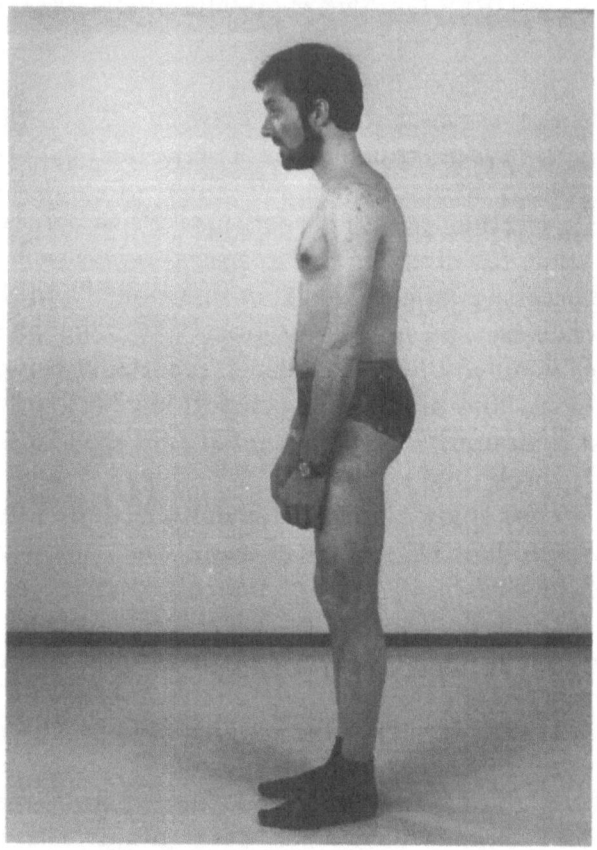

FIGURE 4.1  A, This AS patient has almost complete ankylosis of his spine. The posture is, however, largely unaltered except for a moderately increased cervico-dorsal kyphosis.

segments, but interscapular and cervical pain may also be initial complaints. The back pain of AS usually starts gradually before 40 years of age and varies markedly in severity. Unlike many other (e.g. mechanical) back disorders, it is not relieved by rest[31]. In contrast, a marked improvement of the pain is frequently experienced by moderate exercise[29,35-37]. A feeling of stiffness accompanies the pain, and it is most pronounced in the early morning or late at night[29,31,36,37]. Disturbed sleep is therefore a common complaint[9,31]. The patients will often say that the pain gets them out of bed at night and is ameliorated

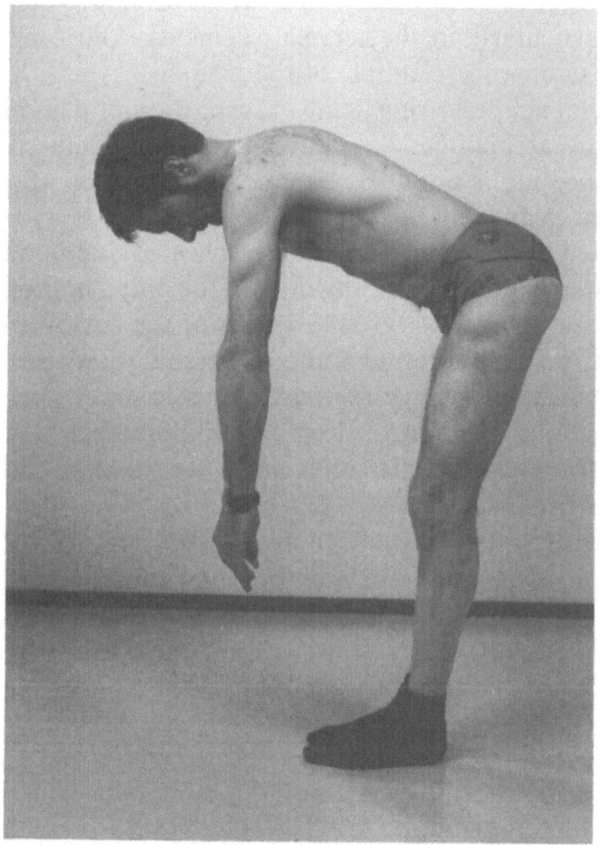

FIGURE 4.1    B, When bending forward, all the movement takes place in the hip joints.

by walking about [37]. The back pain may radiate down the lower extremities, mimicking disc herniation but, unlike this disorder, the radiating pain rarely extends below the knees and is often bilateral, shifting from one extremity to the other[9,38]. As in diseases of the intervertebral disc, the pain in AS may worsen by sneezing or coughing [9,24,38], or by sudden movements[24,38]. Due to involvement of costovertebral joints, pain during deep breathing is frequently observed[28].

Although ossification is a characteristic feature of AS, complete ankylosis with the characteristic 'bamboo spine' as an end stage, is relatively infrequent. The fused spine causes less pain, but is prone to fractures, particularly in the cervical segments, following even relatively mild trauma, for example of the whiplash type[39]. X-ray examination of the back following acute exacerbation of pain and stiffness sometimes reveals changes compatible with spondylodiscitis[40]. Atlanto-axial dislocation is not a frequent complication of AS, but it may result in pareses and can be fatal[41].

Pain located in the anterior part of the chest is common in AS , and may sometimes be the dominating or even the only symptom[25,26,28,31,32]. The chest pain appears to reflect arthritis of the costovertebral, sternoclavicular, manubriosternal and costosternal joints, in addition to enthesopathic lesions at the intercostal muscle insertions. It is worsened by coughing, laughing or deep breath. Sometimes the chest pain is referred to the precordial area and may thus be suspective of coronary heart disease.

Peripheral arthritis may affect up to 20% of the patients with pain, swelling, sometimes erosions and deformities, or fusion[24,26,31,42]. Peripheral arthritis of AS is usually more asymmetric, and more frequently affecting the lower extremities than that of rheumatoid arthritis.

## Systemic features of ankylosing spondylitis

Being a systemic, chronic inflammatory disease, AS may affect many organ systems in addition to the spinal and peripheral joints and insertions of tendons and muscles. The systemic features include fatigue, loss of weight, anaemia, and increased erythrocyte sedimentation rate and acute phase proteins[43,44]. In general, the systemic manifestations of AS are more pronounced in patients with peripheral arthritis and thus less frequent in the typical axial form of the disorder[44].

*Acute anterior uveitis* or iritis, regarded by some as a part of the AS disease complex itself[45], is considered by others to be an independent disorder only statistically associated with AS and HLA-B27[46]. The frequency of iritis in AS is reportedly between 4% and 33%[42,47] and in one study[28] it was found that 2% of the patients with AS presented with iritis while 17% subsequently developed it. The condition may

84

require topical or even systemic treatment with corticosteroids, but the prognosis with respect to vision is generally good.

*Cardiovascular* manifestations include aortitis with subvalvular fibrosis resulting in aortic incompetence and cardiomegaly occurring in some 3–5% of patients with AS and usually after long duration of disease[48]. A significant number of patients coming to aortic valve replacement have AS or a related spondylarthropathy.

Various cardiac conduction disturbances have been reported in from 3% to 33% of patients with AS. The disturbances may vary from a slight prolongation of the P-Q interval on ECG, which is of little clinical significance, to complete atrio-ventricular block[47–49].

*Pulmonary affection*, which involves apical fibrosis of the lungs is occasionally seen, mostly in patients with advanced AS. Mild cases are often symptomless; however, secondary infection may cause severe pulmonary symptoms like cough, dyspnoea, sputum and haemoptysis[50]. Usually the diaphragm provides sufficient pulmonary ventilation, even when the chest has become rigid due to ossification of the joints. However, the 'abdominal' respiration causes increased pressure on the abdominal wall, and some patients with AS may develop and even present with inguinal hernia.

*Reactive (secondary) amyloidosis* occurs in 4–5% of patients with AS, mainly in those with peripheral arthritis and high general disease activity[51]. Although infrequent, amyloidosis is a severe complication of AS, and particularly affection of the kidneys may cause renal failure and early death[51].

*Renal impairment* other than that related to amyloidosis does not appear to be of great importance in AS[52]. However, fatal cases of glomerulopathy associated with AS have been described, and particularly IgA nephropathy may be associated with the seronegative spondylarthropathies[53]. We[54] have noticed abnormalities of the urine sediment compatible with renal affection in 9 out of 78 patients (11%) with AS, mostly in those with high general disease activity and peripheral arthropathy.

Chronic prostatitis appears to occur more frequently in AS than in normal controls[55].

*Neurological symptoms* reported in association with AS include the cauda equina syndrome, focal epilepsy, vertebrobasilar insufficiency and peripheral nerve lesions[56]. As mentioned, atlanto-axial dislocation is not a frequent complication of AS[41].

The systemic nature of AS is also illustrated by its clinical and genetic (i.e. HLA-B27) overlapping with other diseases, like Reiter's disease, psoriasis, inflammatory bowel diseases and Behçet's disease, with sacroiliitis as the common denominator[34].

## Physical signs

At examination, the earliest physical sign of AS is often loss of the lumbar lordosis[24,26,37]. The lateral flexion in the lumbar region is likewise often decreased early in the course of the disease[31,37]. An important clinical sign of AS is restricted anterior flexion of the lumbar spine which can be measured by the modified Schober's test[37,57], and a similar principle can be used to evaluate the lateral mobility in the lumbar region[58]. The total ventral and the dorsal flexion of the lumbar and thoracic spine can be measured using a spondylometer[59]. It should be noted that spinal extension tends to diminish earlier than flexion[37,60]. Limitation of spinal mobility in AS usually affects all planes, which contrasts the finding in disc lesions where lateral flexion is often spared[37,58,61,62]. The restricted spinal mobility in AS also extends to the thoracic region, where measurement of chest expansion reveals reduced values in 41–46% of cases[24,27,37,45,63]. Exact measurements of chest expansion may, however, be difficult, particularly in females.

Clinical evaluation of sacroiliitis may likewise be difficult. Pain elicited by stressing the sacroiliac joints, either directly or indirectly, appears to have little diagnostic significance in general[64]. In one study[65] the only reliable 'sacroiliac sign' was the 'knee to shoulder test' which had a high specificity, but an unfortunate low degree of sensitivity[37].

The physical examination should also consider signs of peripheral arthritis, enthesopathies, and other extra-articular features.

## Laboratory features

The most consistent laboratory abnormality in AS is raised serum IgA[44,66-68], showing that humoral immunity is affected in many patients. Also the complement factor C4 was found to be increased in hospitalized patients, whereas IgG, IgM and C3 were raised in those with accompanying peripheral arthritis[44]. Raised ESR and C-reactive protein indicating high general disease activity was frequently seen, and correlated to peripheral arthritis and levels of IgG, IgA, IgM, C3 and C4[44]. However, none of these abnormalities is diagnostic for AS. The association of AS with HLA-B27 is the subject of another chapter in this book.

## The diagnosis of ankylosing spondylitis

The diagnosis of AS may appear rather easy in advanced and typical cases. The rigid spine and the typical posture of a patient with a fused vertebral column is almost pathognomonic for AS, although patients with diffuse idiopathic skeletal hyperostosis (Forestier's disease) may present with similar features[69,70]. However, in early cases or in cases where the spinal changes are lacking, the diagnosis may be very difficult. In order to meet the need for a proper diagnosis of AS both in clinical practice and for research purposes, several attempts at designing relevant diagnostic criteria have been made[37]. The first criteria were proposed at the Rome Symposium[71] in 1961 (Table 4.1). Both radiological (i.e. sacroiliitis) and clinical criteria were included. The diagnosis of AS should be made when bilateral sacroiliitis and

TABLE 4.1   Criteria (Rome 1961) for diagnosing ankylosing spondylitis[71]

---

*Clinical criteria*
1. Low back pain and stiffness for more than 3 months which is not relieved by rest
2. Pain and stiffness in the thoracic region
3. Limited motion in the lumbar spine
4. Limited chest expansion
5. History or evidence of iritis or its sequelae

*Radiological criterion*
6. X-ray showing bilateral sacroiliac changes characteristic of ankylosing spondylitis (this would exclude bilateral osteoarthrosis of the sacroiliac joints)

The criteria specify that the diagnosis of ankylosing spondylitis should be made when bilateral sacroiliitis and one of five clinical criteria are present, or when four clinical criteria are present.

---

one of five clinical criteria are present, or when four clinical criteria are present. Definite radiological sacroiliitis is thus not obligatory for the diagnosis provided the clinical criteria are met satisfactory. Gofton et al.[72] criticized the Rome criteria in 1966, and consequently a modification was agreed upon at a meeting in New York the same year[73] (Table 4.2). A diagnosis of AS meeting these criteria does require definite radiological signs of sacroiliitis. The clinical criteria put forward by both the Rome and the New York symposia have been criticized, however, as some of the features used are not sensitive enough whereas others lack the necessary specificity. In order to detect cases of AS prior to the development of radiological sacroiliitis, Calin and co-workers[35] proposed a screening test for AS based solely on the clinical history, i.e. five characteristic features of back pain (Table 4.3), which could be useful for two reasons. First, the diagnosis could be made independently of radiological examination which is expensive and means exposure to radiation. Secondly, it could imply early diagnosis, and it is known that evidence of radiological sacroiliitis may take several years to develop. Calin and co-workers[35] found that their screening test for AS had a specificity of 85% and a sensitivity of 95%. The screening test has also been evaluated by van der Linden et al.[62], and found to be only moderately sensitive (38%). It was stated, however, that it could be useful for clinical practice. More evaluation is needed, however, before the usefulness of the screening test may eventually be confirmed. Van der Linden et al.[62] also evaluated the Rome and the New York clinical criteria without finding them satisfactory with respect to sensitivity and specificity. Based on a family and population study, they proposed a small modification of the New York criteria (Table 4.4) in order to improve both qualities.

It is the authors' opinion that radiological sacroiliitis should be maintained a *sine qua non* for the diagnosis of AS as far as clinical, epidemiological and genetic studies are concerned. The concept of 'clinical' AS without radiological changes of the sacroiliac joints, as suggested by others[74,75] should be taken with some caution. Provided future evaluations will confirm that the modified New York criteria (Table 4.4) represent an improvement as compared to the original ones (Table 4.2), the criteria could be used for such research purposes. However, for the early diagnosis of AS, a search for better clinical criteria with respect to both sensitivity and specificity is highly needed.

TABLE 4.2  Clinical criteria (New York, 1966) for ankylosing spondylitis[73]

---

A. *Diagnosis*
1. Limitation of motion of the lumbar spine in all three planes – anterior flexion, lateral flexion, and extension
2. History or the presence of pain at the dorso-lumbar junction or in the lumbar spine
3. Limitation of chest expansion to 1 in. (2.5 cm) or less, measured at the level of the fourth intercostal space

B. *Grading*
Definite AS:
1. Grade 3–4 bilateral sacroiliitis with at least one clinical criterion.
2. Grade 3–4 unilateral or Grade 2 bilateral sacroiliitis with clinical criterion 1 (limitation of back movement in all three planes) or with both clinical criteria 2 and 3 (back pain and limitation of chest expansion)
Probable AS:
Grade 3–4 bilateral sacroiliitis with no clinical criteria

---

TABLE 4.3  Characteristic features of back pain in ankylosing spondylitis[35]

---

1. Age of onset below 40 years
2. Insidious onset
3. Duration greater than 3 months
4. Association with morning stiffness
5. Improvement with exercise

---

Gran[37] recently published an epidemiological survey of the signs and symptoms of AS. Out of 11 clinical symptoms evaluated (Table 4.5) the following five symptoms turned out to have the highest Youden index (sensitivity plus specificity minus 100, see reference 37) and were thus most valuable when sensitivity and specificity are taken together: (1) out of bed at night because of pain; (2) pain not relieved by lying down; (3) a duration of pain of 3 months or more; (4) back pain at night; (5) morning stiffness lasting 30 min or more. Ten different clinical signs (Table 4.6) were also evaluated, and the three signs with the highest Youden index were: (1) reduced lateral mobility; (2) total spinal extension of less than 35° measured by spondylometry; (3) total

89

TABLE 4.4    Modified New York criteria for ankylosing spondylitis[62]

A. *Diagnosis*
1. Clinical criteria
   (a) Low back pain and stiffness for more than 3 months which improves with exercise, but is not relieved by rest.
   (b) Limitation of motion of the lumbar spine in both the sagittal and frontal planes.
   (c) Limitation of chest expansion relative to normal values corrected for age and sex.
2. Radiological criterion
   Sacroiliitis grade $\geqslant 2$ bilaterally or sacroiliitis grade 3–4 unilaterally.

B. *Grading*
1. Definite ankylosing spondylitis if the radiological criterion is associated with at least 1 clinical criterion.
2. Probable ankylosing spondylitis if:
   (a) Three clinical criteria are present.
   (b) The radiological criterion is present without any signs or symptoms satisfying the clinical criteria. (Other causes of sacroiliitis should be considered.)

spinal flexion of 40° or less measured by spondylometry. Based on these five clinical symptoms and three clinical signs, a set of eight clinical diagnostic criteria was suggested (Table 4.7). More than four positive out of these eight criteria yielded a Youden index of 40.4 for the diagnosis of definite AS. No person had 8 positive criteria, and only 2.9% of persons without AS had five or more affirmative responses. All patients with AS gave at least two positive responses. As a tentative conclusion, the relationship between number of diagnostic criteria fulfilled and risk of having AS is given in Table 4.7. We suggest that these clinical diagnostic criteria should be evaluated further and hopefully improved by prospective clinical studies of AS. This would mean that a large number of patients can be excluded from diagnosis on clinical grounds without the use of radiological examination.

The traditional basis for the diagnosis of AS has been a combination of radiological and clinical diagnostic criteria. The radiological features (Figure 4.2) of AS[76,77] are characterized by initial, bilateral, erosive arthritis of the sacroiliac joints. These changes are later followed by ossification, in some cases with bony ankylosis as the terminal

TABLE 4.5 Clinical symptoms in ankylosing spondylitis and in subjects with back pain due to other causes (non-AS)[37]

| Symptom | AS | | Non-AS | | Youden index |
|---|---|---|---|---|---|
| | No. | Sensitivity | No. | Specificity | |
| Out of bed at night | 23 | 65.2 | 308 | 79.2 | 44.2 |
| Pain not relieved by lying down | 20 | 80.0 | 308 | 48.7 | 28.7 |
| Duration of pain 3 months or more | 21 | 71.4 | 308 | 53.6 | 25.0 |
| Back pain at night | 24 | 70.8 | 312 | 53.2 | 24.0 |
| Morning stiffness, 0.5 hours or more | 25 | 64.0 | 311 | 58.8 | 22.8 |
| Age at onset less than 35 y | 26 | 91.7 | 303 | 30.0 | 21.7 |
| Pain or stiffness relieved by exercise | 24 | 75.0 | 311 | 45.3 | 20.3 |
| Radiation of pain to knees only | 18 | 44.4 | 309 | 74.3 | 18.7 |
| Stiffness when lying on a bed | 19 | 47.4 | 274 | 67.2 | 14.6 |
| Age at onset of 40 y or less | 26 | 100.0 | 303 | 6.5 | 6.5 |
| Chronic onset of back pain | 19 | 52.6 | 296 | 50.7 | 3.3 |

stage. Spinal changes are erosions on the anterior corners of the vertebrae, often with sclerosis of the corresponding bone, the so-called 'shining corners', straightening of the anterior vertebral margin – 'squaring', and development of bridging syndesmophytes close to the disc space to form the ultimate 'bamboo spine'. When occurring, the spinal changes of AS are often first seen in the dorsolumbar junction, and X-rays of this part of the spine in addition to the sacroiliac joints may give useful information about the extent of the disease. We[78] and others[79] have described some patients who had typical spinal changes of AS in the dorsolumbar segments, but without concomitant arthritis

TABLE 4.6   Clinical signs in ankylosing spondylitis and in subjects with back pain due to other causes[37]

| Sign | AS No. | Sensitivity | Non-AS No. | Specificity | Youden index |
|---|---|---|---|---|---|
| Reduced lateral mobility | 21 | 52.4 | 309 | 82.1 | 34.5 |
| Spondylometry, extension <35° | 23 | 95.7 | 312 | 36.9 | 32.6 |
| Spondylometry, extension <20° | 23 | 43.5 | 311 | 85.9 | 29.4 |
| Spondylometry flexion <40° | 23 | 26.1 | 312 | 96.8 | 22.9 |
| Schober's test <4 cm | 23 | 30.4 | 315 | 86.3 | 16.7 |
| Flattened lumbar lordosis | 25 | 36.0 | 309 | 80.3 | 16.3 |
| Chest expansion <7 cm | 22 | 63.0 | 297 | 53.2 | 16.2 |
| Chest expansion <2.5 cm | 22 | 9.1 | 297 | 99.7 | 8.8 |
| Knee–shoulder test | 21 | 14.3 | 308 | 89.0 | 3.3 |
| Tenderness over SIJ | 22 | 27.3 | 313 | 67.7 | − 5.0 |

of the sacroiliac joints. Whether these cases represent 'true' AS[80] or a different disease entity[81] can only be verified by prospective follow-up, which is presently being done.

As previously stated, the development of typical radiological features is a late event in AS. The use of radionuclides for scintigraphy

FIGURE 4.2   Top: Radiograph of normal sacroiliac joints. Middle: Erosive phase of bilateral sacroiliitis. Bottom: Terminal stage of sacroiliitis with almost complete bilateral ankylosis in addition to marked ossification of the intervertebral disc. The radiographs were kindly provided by Dr Knut Dale[77].

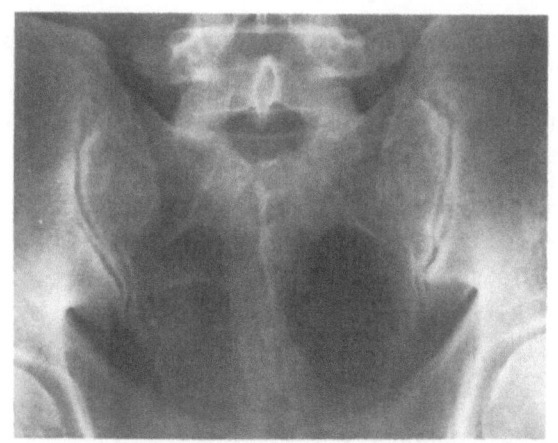

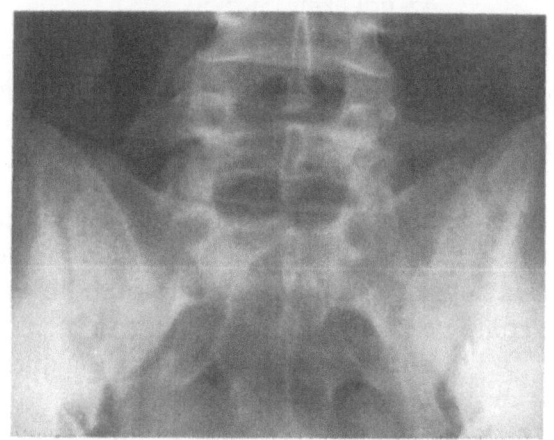

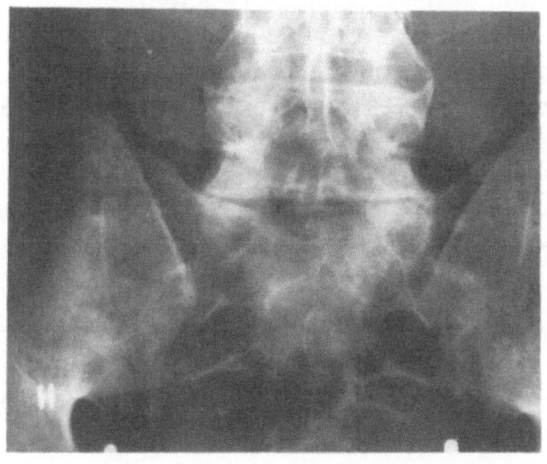

TABLE 4.7   Proposed clinical criteria for AS-relation to disease

---

*Clinical criteria*
1. Out of bed at night because of pain
2. Pain not relieved by lying down
3. Duration of pain 3 months or more
4. Back pain at night
5. Morning stiffness, 0.5 hours or more
6. Reduced lateral spinal mobility
7. Spondylometry, extension < 35°
8. Spondylometry, flexion < 40°

| *Number of criteria present* | *Disease* |
|---|---|
| 0–1 | non-AS |
| 2–3 | AS not likely |
| 4–5 | possible AS |
| 6–7 | probable AS |
| 8 | AS most likely |

---

and quantitative scanning techniques have been used for an earlier diagnosis of AS. However, the specificity of such methods has been questioned[82]. Having an acceptable degree of both sensitivity and specificity[82,83], computed tomography appears to be more promising in this respect. Only future research can answer the question whether magnetic resonance imaging (MRI) will be of help in the early diagnosis of AS. Theoretically, this technique could also provide a quantitative evaluation of the inflammatory activity[83].

Although very sensitive, the diagnostic value of a positive HLA-B27 test for the diagnosis of AS has been questioned[84,85]. However, in a recent population survey of AS in Northern Norway[19] studying subjects between the ages of 20 and 50 years we found that 22% of B27 positive persons complaining of pain or stiffness in the back lasting for at least 4 weeks during the previous year indeed had definite AS according to the New York criteria (Table 4.2). It should also be noted that a negative test for HLA-B27 can be regarded as rather exclusive for AS, as the frequency of AS among HLA-B27 negative persons is 0.2% or less[19,86]. When following up our proposed clinical criteria for AS (Table 4.7), we will also evaluate the usefulness of adding HLA-B27 to the set of criteria.

With regard to differential diagnosis, Forestier's disease[69] or diffuse idiopathic skeletal hyperostosis, has spinal radiological changes which may appear very similar to those of AS, however experienced radiologists can usually observe characteristic differences between the two[70]. More important, the sacroiliac joints are usually radiologically normal in Forestier's disease[70], and furthermore no significant association between Forestier's disease and HLA-B27 is evident[87].

Other differential diagnoses are rheumatic fever when AS has an acute onset, rheumatoid arthritis and other seronegative arthropathies, especially cases with arthritis of the sacroiliac joint, and osteitis condensans ilei in women who have given birth. Also, degenerative, infectious, malignant and metabolic diseases of the locomotor system must sometimes be considered.

Prognosis

The prognosis of AS is generally good[23,42,67]. The discomfort is regarded as most severe in the first 10 years of the disease[23], but on average more than half of the AS patients will be fully employed throughout the disease[23-25,46,88]. With regard to life expectancy, it is a matter of dispute whether the mortality in AS is increased as compared to that of the general population. Some patients with AS certainly have severe systemic manifestation, e.g. cardiac disease[48,49] and renal amyloidosis[51]. However, whether such cases contribute to a shorter life expectancy in AS patients is not agreed upon. Some studies[89,90] conclude with an increased mortality rate in AS, while other workers do not find this[91]. In one study[23] it was found that 13% of the deaths in AS were due to disease-related events such as aortic valve insufficiency, cervical subluxations, respiratory failure and amyloid nephropathy. AS has also been associated with increased risk of several types of cancer[89,91,92], but the patients studied had received radiotherapy. Hypergammaglobulinaemia[93], early peripheral joint involvement and iritis[23] have been associated with severe disease. A less favourable outcome is furthermore expected in patients with involvement of the hip joints[94], and it appears that the functional prognosis of AS is to a large extent dependent on the presence and severity of peripheral arthritis. However, in spite of a favourable

95

prognosis, AS imposes an important and costly health burden on society.

## COMPARISONS BETWEEN MEN AND WOMEN WITH ANKYLOSING SPONDYLITIS

Ankylosing spondylitis (AS) was long considered a disease of the male sex, and studies from 1940 to 1950 [63,95] indicated a male to female ratio of about 16–9:1. Contemporary studies[27,96] which are less frequently quoted by rheumatological textbooks suggested, however, a less pronounced male preponderance of AS, the estimated proportions ranging from 8–5:1.

Most of these observations were based on patient materials derived from hospitals, and were therefore significantly influenced by selection of the various groups. Another reason for the previous underestimation of female AS is the tradition of physicians to accept a diagnosis of AS almost exclusively in males. Moreover, a reluctance to expose female sex organs to X-rays may also have been an important factor for underestimating the diagnosis of AS among females.

Studies of apparently healthy blood donors based on pelvic roentgenograms[17] revealed an exceptionally low degree of male dominance in AS, i.e. a ratio of 2:1. Another striking finding in these studies[17,97] was a 20–25% prevalence of radiological sacroiliitis among blood donors who carried HLA-B27. These investigations have therefore been subjected to much debate as other workers[18] have failed to confirm the observations. Much of the ongoing discussion has focused on the interpretation of arthritic changes in the sacroiliac joints on X-ray.

Furthermore, population surveys, conducted in the 'post-HLA-B27' period[19,98] were unable to confirm the suggestion[17] of an almost equal sex distribution in AS. Based on the epidemiological studies from Hungary[98] and Norway[19], it is still appropriate to claim a significant excess of males among AS patients, and a ratio of approximately 5:1 in favour of this sex appears at present to be most likely. To date, no satisfactory explanation for such a dominance has been offered. Possible effects of pregnancy, oral contraceptives and menopause on disease pathogenesis have not received the same attention in AS as in rheumatoid arthritis. Østensen and co-workers[42] observed no significant effect of child bearing upon the severity and disease activity of AS. The possible influence of sex steroid hormones on the pathogenesis of AS thus remains dubious. In addition, AS has so far not been related to any particular type of occupation which could have explained the unequal sex distribution.

Another putative explanation for underestimation of the female to male proportion in AS, might be differences between the two sexes with regard to clinical expression and disease severity. Even though disputed by some[25,41], several workers have suggested a less severe disease in females as compared to males afflicted by AS[99–101]. Furthermore, some authors have reported a more frequent involvement of both peripheral joints[102,103] and the cervical spine[104] in females with AS, but these observations have also subsequently been refuted by other investigators[105], demonstrating a similar pattern of joint affection in the two sexes. Controversies also exist as to possible differences between men and women concerning age at onset[102,104], degree of spinal radiological changes[100,104,106] and the frequency of associated acute anterior uveitis (AAU)[100,103,105]. No comprehensive explanation for such differences has yet been afforded. A previous suggestion of a reduced prevalence of HLA-B27 in female AS[107] has been contradicted by the vast majority of reports concluding with similar frequencies of this disease susceptibility gene among men and women.

Critical appraisal of the reports dealing with male and female AS appears highly warranted. Unfortunately, most studies suffer from serious methodological problems which to a large extent explain the pronounced discrepancies reported. Some of the observations are hampered by too small patient materials[100,101,104,105], admixture of spondylarthropathies with a different disease outcome than primary AS[104,106], lack of proper definitions of patient materials[101,108,109] and relevant parameters for disease severity[100,101,104,106,108,109] inclusion of 'AS' cases without definite radiological sacroiliitis[100,109] and by a failure to include male patients with AS for reliable comparison when female AS has been subjected to study[100,101,106,108]. The surveys also differ widely in their selection of patients for study. Some of the reports have been based on AS cases selected entirely through specialized hospital departments while other workers have also included patients seen only in the out-patient clinic. One survey[110] presented patient material consisting of cases derived from both the hospital clinic, the corresponding out-patient clinic and from an ongoing population survey of AS in the same region. Clearly, this diversity of patient populations obscures the picture and makes reliable comparison and subsequent valid conclusions extremely difficult.

Our own patient material[110] consisted of 44 females and 82 males, all exhibiting definite radiological sacroiliitis and thereby satisfying the New York criteria[73] for definite AS. Five of the females and 22 of the males were selected through a population survey of AS in Tromsø, Northern Norway[19]. The remaining 39 females and 60 males were patients at the Department of Rheumatology, either hospitalized or seen at the out-patient clinic. Patients with juvenile onset AS (15 years or less), and patients with psoriasis or inflammatory bowel disease were excluded. The mean age of the female patients was 40.5 years as compared to a mean age of 37.4 among males. The mean disease duration was 15.4 years among female AS patients and 14.4 years among the males. The results of this study are shown in Tables 4.8 and 4.9. As shown in Table 4.8 the average age at onset of AS was 24.3 years in females and 23.1 years in males, a difference which did not reach statistical significance. Moreover Table 4.8 shows there was no difference between male and female patients with regard to: initial symptoms; work performance; frequency of peripheral joint involvement and AAU. Table 4.9 indicates that no difference was found

TABLE 4.8   Age at onset, initial symptoms, frequency of work perform-ance, HLA-B27, AAU and peripheral joint involvement in males and females with definite ankylosing spondylitis

| | Age at onset (y) | Frequency of employ-ment (%) | HLA-B27 (%) | AAU (%) | Frequency of peripheral joint involvement (%) | Initial symptom (%) | |
|---|---|---|---|---|---|---|---|
| | | | | | | Lumbar pain | Peripheral arthritis |
| Females | 24.3 | 68.6 | 98.0 | 23.0 | 29.0 | 72.0 | 5.6 |
| Males | 23.1 | 68.6 | 89.0 | 24.0 | 29.0 | 79.7 | 14.5 |
| Total | 23.5 | 68.6 | 95.0 | 24.0 | 29.0 | 77.1 | 11.4 |

TABLE 4.9   Measurements of spinal mobility in men and women with ankylosing spondylitis

|  | Mean chest expansion (cm) | Mean spondylometry, flexion (degrees) | Mean spondylometry extension (degrees) | Schober's test (cm) |
|---|---|---|---|---|
| Females | 4.4 | 36.1 | 12.9 | 2.7 |
| Males | 4.1 | 34.9 | 14.1 | 3.1 |
| Total | 4.2 | 35.3 | 13.7 | 2.9 |

between the two sexes with respect to restriction of spinal mobility and chest expansion.

It is therefore the authors' opinion that when only cases satisfying the New York criteria[73] for definite AS are accepted, no clear-cut differences between male and female cases with AS will emerge with regard to clinical signs and symptoms, disease course, severity, and prognosis.

When it comes to X-ray, it has been suggested that females with AS generally exhibit a less severe and less widespread disease than male patients[14]. No study has yet emerged, claiming a more severe radiological disease appearance among females. Our own experience[111] is compatible with the view that males exhibit more advanced X-ray changes. Unfortunately, very few studies have focused on radiological features of men and women suffering from this disease. This may be due to difficulties in the interpretation of radiological changes of AS. A relatively high degree of both inter- and intraobserver variation in the grading of arthritic changes in the spine and sacroiliac joints has been demonstrated[112].

In our study of 50 females and 82 males with AS[111] the females had less severe arthritic changes in the sacroiliac joints as compared to males. Probably due to the small number of cases studied, the difference did not, however, reach statistical significance. The unacceptably high degree of interobserver variation in the interpretation of radiological sacroiliitis in our study makes it necessary to subject the patient material to careful follow-up to confirm possible sex differences. Furthermore, longitudinal studies possess another advantage by providing an opportunity to investigate the radiological progression of the disease. If possible, such follow-up studies should also employ computerized tomography better to reveal conceivable progressions.

The impression of more advanced X-ray changes in the sacroiliac joints among males was to some extent strengthened by the findings in the spine. The total frequency of radiological involvement of the lumbar spine was thus significantly less in females than in males, 44.2% versus 74.6% respectively. The so-called 'bamboo-spine' was found twice as frequently in males (14.1%) as compared to females (7.0%). The findings indicate that the process of bony ankylosis is less pronounced among female AS patients. As mentioned earlier, the possible influence of female sex hormones and child bearing on the course of AS in females needs to be explored further. Do multipara patients exhibit more or less severe arthritis than nullipara? To what extent is the arthritis in female AS influenced by previous use of oral contraceptive pills? Both questions are yet to be answered.

Another radiological feature of AS is arthritic changes in the pubic symphysis. In AS, these changes seem predominantly to affect female patients. Does pregnancy influence the development of such features?

The impression of a less-severe radiologically expressed disease in women with AS apparently contrasted our finding[110] of a striking similarity in clinical disease expression and severity among the two sexes. A possible explanation may be that the correlations between clinical features and X-ray changes are different in men and women. The apparent discrepancy observed may also indicate that factors other than the arthritic process, as visualized by X-ray may produce clinical signs and symptoms in females with AS.

Future comparisons of this sort should meet the following requirements in order to provide answers to the posted questions: a sufficient number of males and females to permit reliable statistical analyses; the patient must satisfy accepted diagnostic criteria for AS including radiological sacroiliitis; spondyloarthropathic variants other than primary AS should be excluded from the patient materials and studied independently; well-defined criteria for disease severity and prognosis should be employed, and finally the studies should preferably be conducted longitudinally to allow evaluations of disease progression and final disease outcome. Whether or not adult and juvenile AS should be studied separately in such investigations can be debated. The difficulties in the interpretation of radiological changes may to some extent be overcome by applying standard gradings of the changes[76] and by using two or more independent and 'blinded' radiologists. If significant clinical or radiological differences between males and females are demonstrated, the implications regarding diagnosis and treatment should be outlined.

In spite of obviously conflicting views, we tentatively suggest that a diagnosis of AS in a female patient must be suspected on the same clinical grounds as in males. There is, however, substantial evidence to expect a slower progression of radiological changes in the female patient. Thus, clinicians should accept a longer pre-radiological period of AS in females than in males. Based on our own experience, radiological sacroiliitis will develop within 4 and 6 years after onset of symptoms in males and females respectively.

## HOSPITAL VERSUS EPIDEMIOLOGICAL CASES OF ANKYLOSING SPONDYLITIS

Undoubtedly, differences exist between diagnoses established by epidemiologists and those traditionally accepted by physicians employed in clinical medicine. To include a large number of patients, epidemiologists tend to prefer diagnostic criteria of high sensitivity. Often, inevitably, the specificity is subsequently lowered and a significant number of 'false positives' are included. Clinicians are more concerned about achieving a correct diagnosis and appropriate therapeutic regimens for the actual patient, and are reluctant to accept criteria with low specificity. Consequently, using highly specific criteria with lower sensitivity the clinician must risk losing cases with actual AS, i.e. 'false negative' cases. Generally, a broader spectrum of the disease is observed in population surveys, which contrasts the selected severe cases most often referred to hospitals.

The vast majority of studies on AS originate from departments of rheumatology and orthopaedics, hence the radiological and clinical features of the patients may be representative of only a small minority of AS patients. Consequently, the general practitioner receiving his knowledge through published hospital material runs the risk of predicting a less-favourable outcome than the real one. Data obtained through population surveys are usually closer to reality in this respect. Another advantage offered by population studies is the opportunity

101

to study the natural course of the disease, i.e. the disease course run by patients never given appropriate treatment.

In order to address such problems, a population survey was undertaken in Tromsø, Northern Norway in 1979[19]. Altogether 27 cases of definite AS according to the New York criteria[73] were detected and compared clinically[67] and radiologically[113] with patients attending the local and regional hospital. As expected, the epidemiological cases of AS demonstrated significantly less restricted spinal and chest mobility than the hospitalized patients (Table 4.10). Furthermore, a higher frequency of full-time employment was observed in the group of epidemiological patients (89% versus 63% among hospitalized cases). Comparing the two groups for radiological features revealed the same impression, a milder disease among those selected through the population survey. The male hospitalized patients exhibited more severe X-ray changes in the sacroiliac joints than did the epidemiological cases. The female patients admitted to hospital due to AS-related events had more frequently (47.5%) changes in the lumbar spine typical of AS compared to females detected by the population survey (0%).

The main impression gained is thus that AS patients seen in hospitals represent the more severe cases of the disease, both with regard to radiological features and clinical disease expression. On the other hand, localization and type of symptoms, age at onset of AS, frequency of AAU and HLA-B27 appear to be similar in the two groups. These findings do not indicate the presence of different subgroups of primary AS diverging on grounds of clinical disparities. The observations rather speak for a wide spectrum of AS exhibiting different degrees of

TABLE 4.10 Measurements of spinal and chest mobility in patients selected through an epidemiological survey (EPI AS) and those admitted to hospital (HOSP AS)

|  | Mean Schober's test (cm) | Mean spondylometry, flexion (degrees) | Mean spondylometry, extension (degrees) | Mean chest expansion (cm) |
|---|---|---|---|---|
| EPI AS | 3.9 | 45 | 20 | 5.1 |
| HOSP AS | 2.6 | 31 | 15 | 3.6 |

disease severity. Furthermore, better disease outcome than usually accepted can be predicted in AS. This should encourage the physician to earlier diagnosis in order to prescribe appropriate therapeutic regimens. Most frequently, a favourable response to his efforts can be expected.

## References

1. Ott, V. R. (1979). Bechterew's syndrome – a historical review., *Scand. J. Rheumatol.*, Suppl. 32, 6–13
2. Pausanias. Periklet. 1.25.6 ab. 100 A.C. Translated by W. H. S. Jones in The Loeb Classical Library
3. Connor, B. (1695). An extract of a letter from Bernard Connor, M. D. to Sir Charles Walgrave, published in French at Paris. *Philos. Trans. Roy. Soc. London,* **9,** 21–7
4. Kåss, E. (1979). Bechterew's syndrome and allied disorders. *Scand. J. Rheumatol.*, Suppl. 32, 14–5
5. Calin, A. and Marks, S. (1981). Management of ankylosing spondylitis. *Bull. Rheum. Dis.*, **31,** 35–8
6. Kåss, E. (1975). The pathogenesis of ankylosing spondylitis. *Ann. Clin. Res.*, **7,** 237–8
7. Brewerton, D. A., Hart, F. D., Nicholls, A., Caffrey, M., James, D. C. O. and Sturrock, R. D. (1973). Ankylosing spondylitis and HL-A27. *Lancet*, **1,** 904–7
8. Schlosstein, L., Terasaki, P. I., Bluestone, R. and Pearson, C. M. (1973). High association of an HL-A antigen, W27, with ankylosing spondylitis. *N. Engl. J. Med.*, **288,** 704–6
9. Iversen, P. F. (1948). Spondylarthritis anchylopoetica (morbus Bechterew). *Nord. Med.*, **39,** 1707–9
10. de Blecourt, J. J., Polman, A. and de Blecourt-Meindersma, T. (1961). Hereditary factors in rheumatoid arthritis and ankylosing spondylitis. *Ann. Rheum. Dis.*, **20,** 215–20
11. Rogoff, B. and Freyberg, R. H. (1949). The familiar incidence of rheumatoid spondylitis. *Ann. Rheum. Dis.*, **8,** 139–42
12. Hersh, A. H., Stecher, R. M., Solomon, W. M., Wolpaw, R. and Hauser, H. (1950). Heredity in ankylosing spondylitis. A study of fifty families. *Am. J. Hum. Genet.*, **2,** 391–408
13. Moesmann, G. (1960). Hereditary and exogenous etiological factors in ankylosing spondylitis. *Acta Rheum. Scand.*, **6,** 144–50
14. Eastmond, C. J. and Woodrow, J. C. (1977). Discordance for ankylosing spondylitis in monozygotic twins. *Ann. Rheum. Dis.*, **36,** 360–4
15. Ebringer, A. (1979). Ankylosing spondylitis, immune-response genes and molecular mimicry. *Lancet*, **2,** 1186
16. Seager, K., Bashir, H. V., Geczy, A. F., Edmonds, J. and deVere-Tyndall, A. (1979). Evidence for a specific B-27-associated cell surface marker on lymphocytes of patients with ankylosing spondylitis. *Nature*, **277,** 68–70
17. Calin, A. and Fries, J. F. (1975). The striking prevalence of ankylosing spondylitis in 'healthy' W27 positive males and females. *N. Engl. J. Med.*, **293,** 835–9

18. Christiansen, F. T., Hawkins, B. R., Dawkins, R. L., Owen, E. T. and Potter, R. M. (1979). The prevalence of ankylosing spondylitis among B27 positive normal individuals – a reassessment. *J. Rheumatol.*, **6**, 713–18

19. Gran, J. T., Husby, G. and Hordvik, M. (1985). Prevalence of ankylosing spondylitis in males and females in young middle-aged population in Tromsø, Northern Norway. *Ann. Rheum. Dis.*, **44**, 359–67

20. Fassbender, H. G. (1979). Pathological aspects and findings of Bechterew's syndrome and osteoarthropathia psoriatica. *Scand. J. Rheumatol.*, Suppl. 32, 50–8

21. Ball, J. (1979). Articular pathology of ankylosing spondylitis. *Clin. Orthop,*, **143**, 30–7

22. Jacobs, J. C. (1983). Spondylarthritis and enthesopathy. *Arch. Intern. Med.,* **143**, 103–7

23. Carette, S., Graham, D., Little, H., Rubenstein, J. and Rosen, P. (1983).The natural disease course of ankylosing spondylitis. *Arthritis Rheum.*, **26**, 186–90

24. Rosen, P. S. and Graham, D. C. (1962). Ankylosing (Strümpell-Marie) spondylitis. *Arch. Interamer. Rheumatol.*, **5**, 158–233

25. Wilkinson M. and Bywaters, E. G. L. (1958). Clinical features and course of ankylosing spondylitis. As seen in a follow-up 222 Hospital Referred Cases. *Ann. Rheum. Dis.*, **17**, 209–28

26. Polley, H. F. and Slocomb, C. H. (1947). Rheumatoid spondylitis: A study of 1035 cases. *Ann. Intern. Med.*, **26**, 240–9.

27. Simpson, N. R. W. and Stevenson, C. J. (1949). An analysis of 200 cases of ankylosing spondylitis. *Br. Med. J.*, **1**, 214–16

28. Sigler, J. W., Bluhm, G. B., Duncan, H. and Ensign, D. C. (1971). Clinical features of ankylosing spondylitis. *Clin. Orthop. Rel. Res.*, **74**, 14–19.

29. Møller, P., Vinje, O. and Kåss, E. (1982). How does Bechterew's syndrome (ankylosing spondylitis) start? *Scand. J. Rheumatol.*, **12**, 289–98

30. Adler, E. and Carmon, A. (1961). Ankylosing Spondylitis – review of 115 cases. *Acta. Rheum. Scand.*, **7**, 219–32

31. Kåss, E. (1968). Diagnostic criteria in spondylarthritis ankylopoietica. *Acta. Rheum. Scand.*, **14**, 197–209

32. Good, A. E. and Arbor, A. (1963). The chest pain of ankylosing spondylitis. Its place in the differential diagnosis of heart pain. *Ann. Intern. Med.*, **58**, 926–37

33. Reitan, H. (1965). Some features of mb. Bechterew by X-ray examination. *Acta Rheum. Scand.* **11**, 15–18

34. Moll, J. M. H., Haslock, J., Macrae, I. F. and Wright, V. (1974). Associations between ankylosing spondylitis, psoriatic arthritis, Reiter's disease, the intestinal arthropathies, and Behcet's syndrome. *Medicine,* **53**, 343–64

35. Calin, A., Porta, J., Fries, J. F. and Schurman, D. J. (1977). Clinical history as a screening test for ankylosing spondylitis. *J. Am. Med. Assoc.*, **237**, 2613–14

36. Christiansen, F. T., Owen, E. T., Dawkins, R. L. and Hanrahan, P. (1977). Symptoms and signs among relatives of patients with HLA-B27 ankylosing spondylitis: Correlation between back pain, spinal movement, sacroiliitis and HLA-antigens. *J. Rheumatol.* Suppl. 3, 11–17

37. Gran, J. T. (1985). An epidemiological survey of the signs and symptoms of ankylosing spondylitis. *Clin. Rheum.*, **4**, 161–9

38. Tandberg, A. (1950) Initial symptoms in spondylarthritis ankylopoietica. *Rheumatism,* **6**, 127–32

39. Hunter, T. and Dubo, H. (1975) Spinal fractures complicating ankylosing spondylitis. *Ann. Intern. Med.*, **88**, 546–9
40. Sutherland, R. I. L. and Matheson, D. (1975). Inflammatory involvement of vertebrae in ankylosing spondylitis. *J. Rheumatol.*, **2**, 296–302
41. Spencer, D. G., Park, W. M., Dick, H. M., Papazoglou, S. N. and Buchanan, W. W. (1979). Radiological manifestations in 200 patients with ankylosing spondylitis: Correlation with clinical features and HLA-B27. *J. Rheumatol.*, **6**, 305–15
42. Østensen, M., Romberg, Ø. and Husby, G. (1982). Ankylosing spondylitis and motherhood. *Arthr. Rheum.*, **25**, 140–3
43. Hart, F. D. (1968). The stiff aching back. The differential diagnosis of ankylosing spondylitis. *Lancet*, **1**, 740–2
44. Vinje, O., Møller, P. and Mellbye, O. J. (1984). Immunological parameters and acute-phase reactants in patients with Bechterew's syndrome (ankylosing spondylitis) and their relatives. *Clin. Rheumatol.*, **3**, 501–14
45. Møller, P., Vinje, O., Dale, K., Berg, K. and Kåss, E. (1984). Family studies in Bechterew's syndrome (ankylosing spondylitis). *Scand. J. Rheumatol.*, **13**, 1–10
46. Ebringer, R., Cawdell, D. and Ebringer, A. (1979). Klebsiella pneumoniae and acute anterior uveitis in ankylosing spondylitis. *Br. Med. J.*, **1**, 383
47. Parr, L. J. A., White, P. and Shipton, E. (1951). Some observations on 100 cases of ankylosing spondylitis. *Med. J. Aust.*, **2**, 544–8
48. Bachmann, F. and Hart, W. (1976) Kardiovaskuläre Komplikationen bei Spondylitis ankylosans (Morbus Bechterew). *Dtsch. Med. Wochenschr.*, **101**, 864–6
49. Bergfeldt, L., Edhag, O. and Vallin, H. (1982). Cardiac conduction disturbances, an underestimated manifestation in ankylosing spondylitis. *Acta Med. Scand.*, **212**, 217–23.
50. Anonymous. (1971). The lungs in ankylosing spondylitis. *Br. Med. J.*, **3**, 492
51. Husby, G. (1980). Amyloidosis in ankylosing spondylitis. *Scand. J. Rheumatol.*, Suppl. 32, 67–70
52. Calin, A. (1975). Renal glomerular function in ankylosing spondylitis. *Scand. J. Rheumatol.*, **4**, 241–2
53. Jennette, J. C., Ferguson, A. L., Moore, M. A. *et al.* (1982). IgA nephropathy associated with seronegative spondylarthropathies. *Arthritis Rheum.*, **25**, 144–9
54. Omdal, R. and Husby, G. (1986). Renal affection in ankylosing spondylitis and psoriatic arthropathy? *Clin. Rheumatol.*, **6**, 74–9
55. Mason, R. M., Murray, R. S., Oates, J. K. *et al.* (1958). Prostatitis and ankylosing spondylitis. *Br. Med. J.*, **1**, 748–51
56. Thomas, J., Kendall, M. J. and Whitfield, A. G. W. (1974). Nervous system involvement in ankylosing spondylitis. *Br. Med. J.*, **1**, 148–50
57. Macrae, I. F. and Wright, V. (1969). Measurement of back movement. *Ann. Rheum. Dis.*, **28**, 584–91
58. Moll, J. M. H. and Wright, V. (1971). Normal range of spinal mobility: An objective clinical study. *Ann. Rheum. Dis.*, **30**, 381–6
59. Hart, F. D., Strickland, C. and Cliffe, P. (1974). Measurement of spinal mobility. *Ann. Rheum. Dis.*, **33**, 136–9
60. Sturrock, R. D., Wojtulewski, J. A. and Dudley-Hart. F. (1973). Spondylometry in a normal population and in ankylosing spondylitis. *Rheumatol. Rehabil.*, **12**, 135–42

61. Cheshire, D. J. E. and Nichols, P. J. R. (1955). The early stages of ankylosing spondylitis. *Rheumatism,* **11,** 79–82
62. Van der Linden, S., Valkenburg, H. A. and Cats, A. (1984). Evaluation of diagnostic criteria for ankylosing spondylitis. A proposal for modification of the New York Criteria. *Arthritis Rheum.,* **27,** 361–8
63. Graham, W. and Orgryzlo, M. A. (1974). Ankylosing (Marie–Strümpell) spondylitis. (An analysis of 100 cases). *Can. Med. Assoc. J.,* **57,** 16–21
64. Russel, A. S., Maksymowych, W. and LeClercq, S. (1981). Clinical examination of the sacroiliac joints: a prospective study. *Arthritis Rheum.,* **24,** 1575–7
65. Rudge, S. R., Swannell, A. J., Rose, D. H. and Todd, J. H. (1982). The clinical assessment of sacroiliac joint involvement in ankylosing spondylitis. *Rheumatol. Rehabil.,* **21,** 15–20
66. Kinzella, T. D., Spinoza, L. and Vaseg, F. B. (1975). Serum complement and immunoglobulin levels in sporadic and familial ankylosing spondylitis. *J. Rheumatol.,* **2,** 308–13
67. Gran, J. T. and Husby, G. (1984). Ankylosing spondylitis. A comparative study of patients found in an epidemiological survey, and those admitted to a Department of Rheumatology. *J. Rheumatol.,* **11,** 788–93
68. Østensen, M. (1984). The influence of pregnancy on blood parameters in patients with rheumatic disease. A prospective study. *Scand. J. Rheumatol.,* **13,** 203–8
69. Forestier, J. and Lagier, R. (1971). Ankylosing hyperostosis of the spine. *Clin. Orthop.,* **74,** 65–83
70. Resnick, D., Shapiro, R. F., Wiesner, K. B., Niwayama, G., Utsinger, P. D. and Shaul, S. R. (1978). Diffuse idiopathic skeletal hyperostosis (DISH) (Ankylosing hyperostosis of Forestier and Rotes-Querol). *Semin. Arthritis Rheum.,* **7,** 153–87
71. Kellgren, J. H. and Jeffrey, M. R. (eds.) (1963). *The Epidemiology of Chronic Rheumatism.* Vol. 1, pp. 326–7 (Oxford: Blackwell Scientific)
72. Gofton, J. P., Lawrence, J. S., Bennett, P. H. and Burch, T. A. (1966). Sacroiliitis in eight populations. *Ann. Rheum. Dis.,* **25,** 528–33
73. Bennet, P. H. and Burch, T. A. (eds.) (1968). *Population Studies of the Rheumatic Diseases,* pp. 456–7. (Amsterdam: Excerpta Medica)
74. Kahn, M. A., van der Linden, S. J., Kushner, I., Valkenburg, H. A. and Cats, A. (1985). Spondylitic disease without radiologic evidence of sacroiliitis in relatives of HLA-B27 positive ankylosing spondylitis patients. *Arthritis Rheum.,* **28,** 40–3
75. Anonymous (1985). Spondylitis: Time for a new name and a new approach to diagnosis. *Lancet,* **2,** 479–81
76. Dale, K. (1979). Radiographic changes of the spine in Bechterew's syndrome and allied disorders. *Scand. J. Rheumatol.,* Suppl. 32, 103–9
77. Dale, K. (1980). Radiographic grading of sacroiliitis in Bechterew's syndrome and allied disorders. *Scand. J. Rheumatol.,* Suppl. 32, 92–7
78. Gran, J. T., Husby, G. and Hordvik, M. (1985). Spinal ankylosing spondylitis: A variant form of ankylosing spondylitis, or a distinct disease entity? *Ann. Rheum. Dis.,* **44,** 368–71
79. Jajic, I., Furst, Z. and Vuksic, B. (1982). Spondylitis erosiva: report on 9 patients. *Ann. Rheum. Dis.,* **41,** 237–41
80. Calin, A. (1979). Ankylosing spondylitis sine sacroiliitis. *Arthritis. Rheum.,* **22,** 303–4

81. Courtois, C., Fallet, G. H., Vischer, T. L. and Wettstein, P. (1980). Erosive spondylopathy. *Ann. Rheum. Dis.*, **39**, 462–8
82. Taggart, A. J., Desai, S. M., Iveson, J. M. and Verow, P. W. (1984). Computerized tomography of the sacro-iliac joints in the diagnosis of sacro-iliitis. *Br. J. Rheumatol.*, **23**, 258–66
83. Buckland-Wright, J. C. (1983). Advances in the radiological assessment of rheumatoid arthritis. *Br. J. Rheumatol.*, Suppl. 22, 34–43
84. Esdaile, J. M., Dwosh, I. L., Urowitz, M. B., Smythe, H. A. and Falk, J. (1977). HLA-B27 in rheumatoid factor – negative polyarthritis. *Ann. Intern. Med.*, **86**, 699–702
85. Calin, A. (1980). HLA-B27: To type or not to type. *Ann. Intern. Med.*, **92**, 208–11
86. Hawkins, B. R., Dawkins, R. L., Christiansen, F. T. and Zilko, P. J. (1981). Use of the B27 test in the diagnosis of ankylosing spondylitis: A statistical evaluation. *Arthritis Rheum.*, **24**, 743–6
87. Shapiro, R. F., Utsinger, P. D. and Wiesner, K. B. (1976). The association of HLA-B27 with Forestier's disease (vertebral ankylosing hyperostosis). *J. Rheumatol.*, **3**, 4–8
88. Vobecky, J., Lussier, A. and Munan, L. (1974). Rheumatoid arthritis and ankylosing spondylitis in an ethnically homogeneous population: Familial distribution of complaints. *J. Chron. Dis.*, **27**, 413–25
89. Radford, E. P., Doll, R. and Smith, P. G. (1977). Mortality among patients with ankylosing spondylitis not given X-ray therapy. *N. Engl. J. Med.*, **297**, 572–6
90. Khan, M. A., Khan, M. K. and Kushner, I. (1981). Survival among patients with ankylosing spondylitis: a life-table analysis. *J. Rheumatol.*, **8**, 86–90
91. Kaprove, R. E., Little, A. H., Graham, D. C. and Rosen, P. S. (1980). Ankylosing spondylitis. Survival in men with and without radiotherapy. *Arthritis Rheum.*, **23**, 57–61
92. Brown, W. M. C. and Doll, R. (1965). Mortality from cancer and other causes after radiotherapy for ankylosing spondylitis. *Br. Med. J.*, **2**, 1327–32
93. Lehtinen, K. (1982). The mortality and causes of death of patients with 'hypergamma' type of ankylosing spondylitis. *Scand. J. Rheumatol.*, **12**, 3–4
94. Garcia-Morteo, O., Maldonado-Cocco, J. A., Suárez-Almazor, M. E. and Garay, E. (1983). Ankylosing spondylitis of juvenile onset: comparison with adult onset disease. *Scand. J. Rheumatol.*, **12**, 246–8
95. West, H. F. (1949). The aetiology of ankylosing spondylitis. *Ann. Rheum. Dis.*, **8**, 143–8
96. Fletcher, E. (1944). Ankylosing spondylitis. *Lancet*, **1**, 754–6
97. Cohen, L. M., Mittal, K. K., Schmid, F. R., Rogers, L. F. and Cohen, K. L. (1976). Increased risk for spondylitis stigmata in apparently healthy HLA-B27 men. *Ann. Intern. Med.*, **84**, 1–7
98. Gömör, B., Gyodi, E. and Bakos, L. (1977). Distribution of HLA-B27 and ankylosing spondylitis in the Hungarian population. *J. Rheumatol.*, Suppl. 3, 33–5
99. Tyson, T. L., Thomson, W. A. L. and Ragan, C. (1953). Marie Strümpell spondylitis in women. *Ann. Rheum. Dis.*, **12**, 40–2
100. Hill, H. F. H., Hill, A. G. S. and Bodmer, J. G. (1976). Clinical diagnosis of ankylosing spondylitis in women and relation to presence of HLA-B27. *Ann. Rheum. Dis.*, **35**, 267–70

101. Jeannet, M., Saudan, Y. and Bitter, T. (1975). HL-A27 in female patients with ankylosing spondylitis. *Tissue Antigens,* **6,** 262–4
102. Goodman, C. E., Lange, R. K., Waxman, J. and Weis, T. E. (1980). Ankylosing spondylitis in women. *Arch. Phys. Med. Rehabil.,* **61,** 167–70
103. Molony, J. and Thompson, R. (1979). Ankylosing spondylitis in women. A review of 8 cases. *J. Irish Med. Assoc.,* **72,** 236–7
104. Resnick, D., Dwosh, I. L., Goergen, T. G., Shapiro, R. T., Utsinger, P. D., Wiesner, K. B. and Bryan, B. L. (1976). Clinical and radiographic abnormalities in ankylosing spondylitis: A comparison of men and women. *Diagn. Radiol.,* **119,** 293–7
105. Marks, S. H., Barnett, M. and Calin, A. (1983). Ankylosing spondylitis in women and men: a case control study. *J. Rheumatol.,* **10,** 624–8
106. Hart, F. D. and Robinson, K. C. (1959). Ankylosing spondylitis in women. *Ann. Rheum. Dis.,* **18,** 15–23
107 Swezey, R. L., Zucker, L. M. and Terasaki, P. I. (1974). Reduced prevalence of HL-A antigen W27 in black females with ankylosing spondylitis. *J. Rheumatol.,* **1,** 260–2
108. Pohl, W. and Treiber, W. (1962). Morbus Bechterew beim weiblichen Geschlecht. *Münch. Med. Wochenschr.,* **104,** 674–8
109. Jevleva, L. V., Akimova, T. F. and Mylov, N. M. (1984). Bechterew's disease in women. *Scand. J. Rheumatol.,* Suppl. 52, 13–15
110. Gran, J. T., Østensen, M. and Husby, G. (1985). A clinical comparison between males and females with ankylosing spondylitis. *J. Rheumatol.,* **12,** 126–9
111. Gran, J. T., Husby G., Hordvik, M., Størmer, J. and Romberg-Andersen, Ø. (1984). Radiological changes in men and women with ankylosing spondylitis. *Ann. Rheum. Dis.,* **43,** 570–5
112. Hollingsworth, P. N., Cheak, P. S., Dawkins, R. L., Owen, E. T., Calin, A. and Wood, P. H. N. (1983). Observer variation in grading sacroiliac radiographs in HLA-B27 positive individuals. *J. Rheumatol.,* **2,** 247–54
113. Gran, J. T., Hordvik, M. and Husby, G. (1984). Roentgenological features of ankylosing spondylitis. A comparison between patients attending hospital and cases selected through an epidemiological survey. *Clin. Rheumatol.,* **3,** 467–72

# 5

# THE ONSET, EVOLUTION AND FINAL STAGES OF JUVENILE ANKYLOSING SPONDYLITIS ARE DIFFERENT FROM THOSE OF ADULT ANKYLOSING SPONDYLITIS

*J. JIMENEZ and G. MINTZ*

---

Juvenile-onset ankylosing spondylitis is a disease of unknown aetiology that affects primarily males under 16 years of age. It is characterized by early peripheral arthritis of the lower extremities and late onset inflammatory lumbar pain[1-5]. Of reported cases, 90% are B27+[1,5] and 20% have acute iridocyclitis[3,4]. These children are negative for rheumatoid factor and ANA. While sacroiliitis may be found as early as the first year, it may evolve as late as 12 years after onset of peripheral arthritis. Additional features include low-grade fever, family aggregation, and a benign evolution on long-term follow-up[1,5-11].

There are two studies that compare juvenile-onset and adult-onset ankylosing spondylitis. In the report by Marks *et al.*[11] of 22 patients followed for 13 years, the juveniles had more peripheral arthritis and more hip disease but the functional outcome and prognosis were the same for both groups. The other report by Garcia-Morteo *et al.*[7] compares 24 juveniles with 71 adults followed for an average of 15 years. There was a slightly higher female frequency in the juveniles who had more peripheral arthritis and a poorer final functional outcome because of progressive hip involvement.

With the purpose of better defining the possible similarities and differences between juvenile-onset and adult-onset AS, we studied a group of patients with onset before age 16 and compared them with a group of patients whose disease began after that age, with an average duration of illness of 20 years.

## MATERIAL AND METHODS

Of 103 patients with AS who attend our outpatient clinic, 22 were juveniles. The onset of disease was established by reviewing the records from other hospitals in the Centro Medico Nacional where the patients had been originally admitted: the Hospital for Orthopaedic Surgery, the Paediatric Hospital and the Cardiology Hospital. When the patients reached 16 years of age, they were referred to our Department. From previous hospital records, we were able to document signs and symptoms of the initial clinical presentation as well as laboratory studies, therapy and evolution of disease.

Functional class was judged by 2 grades: (1) working or attending school or (2) unable to work or attend school. All patients were seen by an ophthalmologist. The following laboratory examinations were performed: complete blood count, Westergren erythrocyte sedimentation rate, rheumatoid factor (Waaler Rose), antinuclear antibodies (immunofluorescence) and HLA-B27. Radiological studies of the entire spine, pelvis and selected joints were done and graded by independent observers as Class I, only sacroiliitis, Class II, sacroiliitis plus squaring of vertebral bodies, and Class III, ankylosis of sacroiliac joints plus ankylosis of the spine.

The control group, matched by sex and duration of disease, included a group of 22 patients with disease onset after age 16. These patients were studied in the same manner as the juveniles. All patients fulfilled the New York diagnostic criteria for AS[12]. The Students' *t* test was used for statistical analysis of the results.

RESULTS

In the juvenile group, there were 20 males and two females. The average age of onset was 10 years (range 6–15) and the average duration of disease was 20 years. In the adult group, there were 19 males and three females. The average age of onset was 27 years (range 17–44) and the duration of disease averaged 20.8 years. In the juvenile group 20 patients (91%) were HLA-B27 + while 19 (86%) adults were HLA-B27 +.

## Mode of onset

Both groups had a high frequency of peripheral arthritis (Table 5.1) but the knees and ankles were significantly more often involved in the juveniles. Both knees were swollen in 16 juvenile cases and both ankles in five. Hips were involved with the same frequency in both groups but inflammatory low back pain was found in only two of the juveniles as compared with 17 adults. A febrile course was noted in 12 juveniles but in only one adult. Temperatures were usually above 39°C in the evenings, returning to normal at night or in the early morning. These febrile episodes lasted 6 to 8 weeks with occasional intervals of 2 or 3 days of normal temperatures. There were no signs of other organ involvement, no acute anterior uveitis, and blood and other cultures proved to be negative. Laboratory findings included normochromic anaemia, leukocytosis (12 000–18 000) and hypergammaglobulin-aemia which were present at onset as well as during exacerbations.

## Treatment

At onset, all juveniles were hospitalized and treated with aspirin 3 g daily, phenylbutazone 300 mg daily, or indomethacin 75 mg daily. The fever subsided promptly within 7 to 10 days. Persistent peripheral arthritis required 7.5–15 mg of prednisone daily in 10 patients, for varying periods of time and up to one year, after which all patients were asymptomatic and therapy was discontinued.

TABLE 5.1 Clinical and laboratory findings at onset

| Ankylosing spondylitis | No. | Peripheral arthritis | Knees | Ankles | Hips | Lumbar pain | Fever | Haemo- globin <12g | WBC >12 000 | Hyper- gamma globulin- aemia |
|---|---|---|---|---|---|---|---|---|---|---|
| Juvenile onset | 22 | 22 (100%) | 21 (91%) | 15 (68%) | 9 (41%) | 2 (9%) | 12 (55%) | 7 (32%) | 7 (32%) | 7 (32%) |
| Adult onset | 22 | 20 (91%) | 11 (50%) | 7 (32%) | 9 (41%) | 17 (77%) | 1 (4%) | 4 (18%) | 2 (9%) | 5 (23%) |
|  |  | ns | $p<0.01$ | $p<0.03$ | ns | $p<0.001$ | $p<0.001$ | ns | ns | ns |

Table 5.2 Evolution

| Ankylosing spondylitis | No. | Episodic | Chronic | Uveitis | Fever | Functional Class I | Class II |
|---|---|---|---|---|---|---|---|
| Juvenile onset | 22 | 20 (91%) | 2 (9%) | 5 (23%) | 0 | 16 (73%) | 6 (27%) |
| Adult onset | 22 | 7 (32%) | 15 (68%) | 7 (32%) | 0 | 12 (55%) | 10 (45%) |
|  |  | $<0.001$ | $<0.001$ | ns | ns | ns | ns |

## Evolution

The course of the disease was episodic in 20 juveniles (Table 5.2). Reactivation of disease occurred usually after 2 to 5 years of the initial episode. However, there was one patient with peripheral arthritis at age 11 that lasted for 9 months after which he remained asymptomatic until age 33 when he developed acute anterior uveitis, low back pain and radiologic evidence of sacroiliitis. Uveitis and sacroiliitis appeared in four other cases during exacerbations. Two patients had three and five exacerbations of peripheral arthritis before inflammatory back pain appeared. In contrast, only seven adult patients had an episodic clinical course and most of them developed the typical chronic evolution of back pain with intermittent periods of peripheral arthritis.

On final functional assessment, 16 (73%) of the juveniles and 12 (54%) of the adults were working normally. Invalidity was primarily due to hip disease in both groups with five juveniles and four adults requiring total hip prosthesis. The final radiographic staging revealed that 55% of the juveniles had only sacroiliitis while 82% of the adults had both sacroiliac and vertebral ankylosis (Table 5.3).

## DISCUSSION

All patients fulfilled the diagnostic[12] and clinical criteria for ankylosing spondylitis. Of the total group of 103 patients, the female/male ratio was 1:5, similar to other reports[13,14]. Disease began before age 16 in 21%, slightly more frequent than the 10–15% reported in Caucasian

Table 5.3   Final radiological stage*

| Ankylosing spondylitis | GI | GII | GIII |
|---|---|---|---|
| Juvenile onset | 12 (55%) | 2 (9%) | 8 (36%) |
| Adult onset | 4 (18%) | 0 | 18 (82%) |
|  | $p < 0.001$ |  | $p < 0.03$ |

*See text for radiologic staging criteria

populations[8,9,15–17]. In our juveniles there was a male predominance as described by others[1–5,9,11] except for one report[7].

The onset of juvenile AS with fever has been previously reported[4,8–10] but had not been characterized and most descriptions[1–3,6,7,11,13–16] do not mention this symptom. Fever up to 39° and 40°C in a quotidian pattern was present in our patients. Fever was preceded by chills and followed by profuse perspiration, lasting from 7 days to 2 months. The pattern of arthritis was oligoarticular (1–4 joints), usually symmetrical and affecting primarily the knees or ankles. It was accompanied by anaemia, leukocytosis, hypergammaglobulinaemia and loss of weight so that differentiation from Still's disease was often difficult. However, the lack of hepatosplenomegaly, adenopathy, rash, and the male predominance together with a positive HLA-B27 rule out this diagnosis. On the other hand, a firm diagnosis of ankylosing spondylitis of childhood was impossible during the initial episode in the absence of back pain, uveitis or radiographic sacroiliac changes. The intermittent evolution of juvenile-onset AS has been previously suggested[4,8] and our series confirms the finding of bouts of arthritis lasting a few months to a year only to recur usually 2 to 5 years later, but sometimes even 20 years after the original episode. During these recurrences low back pain and uveitis appeared and made the diagnosis of AS possible. In contrast, only seven adults had an episodic evolution; they all developed early low back pain which became persistent with intermittent bouts of peripheral arthritis.

The frequency of acute anterior uveitis during the 20 years of evolution was similar in both groups. Invalidity was mainly due to hip disease, as reported by others[1–3,7,8,11,14,15]. However, the functional status after 20 years of disease was better in our juveniles than in the adults. This finding is similar to previous reports[11] but different from results of Garcia Morteo[7] where 100% of patients had limitation. Surgical hip replacement was needed with the same frequency in juveniles as in adults, a frequency comparable to that reported in adult series[18–20]. After 20 years of disease, radiological grading disclosed the juveniles had less ankylosis than adults, a finding confirmed by previous reports[9,21]. Finally, the diagnosis of juvenile ankylosing spondylitis during the initial episode may be difficult in the absence of back pain, uveitis or radiological sacroiliitis and may be suspected only if the HLA-B27 test is positive.

# References

1. Schaller, J. G. (1977) Juvenile rheumatoid arthritis. *Arthritis Rheum.*, **20** (Suppl.). 165–70
2. Schaller, J. G. (1979). The seronegative spondyloarthropathies of childhood. *Clin. Orthop. Related Res.*, **143**, 76–83
3. Ansell, B. M. (1977). Juvenile chronic polyarthritis. *Arthritis Rheum.*, **20** (Suppl.), 176–80
4. Ansell, B. M. (1980). Juvenile chronic arthritis. In Aplex, J. (ed.) *Rheumatic Disorders in Childhood*, pp. 87–151 (London: Butterworths)
5. Calabro, J. J., Gordon, R. D. and Miller, K. I. (1979). Bechterew's syndrome in children: diagnostic criteria. *Scand. J. Rheumatol.*, **32** (Suppl.), 45–6
6. Calabro, J. J. (1979). Juvenile rheumatoid arthritis. In McCarty, D. J. (ed.) *Arthritis and Allied Conditions*. 9th Edn, pp. 591–601. (Philadelphia: Lea & Febiger)
7. Garcia-Morteo, O., Maldonado-Coco, J. A., Suarez-Almazor, M. E. and Garay, E. (1983). Ankylosing spondylitis of juvenile onset: comparison with adult onset disease. *Scand. J. Rheumatol.*, **12**, 246–8
8. Schaller, J., Bitnum, S. and Wedgwood, R. J. (1969). Ankylosing spondylitis with childhood onset. *J. Pediatr.*, **74**, 505–16
9. Ladd, J. R., Cassidy, J. T. and Martel, W. (1971). Juvenile ankylosing spondylitis. *Arthritis Rheum.*, **14**, 579–90
10. Hart, F. D. (1980). Clinical features and complications. In Moll, J. M. H. (ed.) *Ankylosing Spondylitis*, pp. 52–68 (Edinburgh: Churchill Livingstone)
11. Marks, S. H., Berrett, M. and Calin, A. (1982). A case control study of juvenile and adult onset ankylosing spondylitis. *J. Rheumatol.*, **19**, 739–41
12. Bennett, P. H., Bremner, W. J., Bywaters, E. G. L, Calabro, J. J., McEwen, C. and Martel, W. (1968). Report from the subcommittee on Diagnostic Criteria for Ankylosing Spondylitis. Population Studies of the Rheumatic Diseases. Bennet, P. H. and Wood, P. H. N. (eds.) pp. 4546–70. (Amsterdam: Excerpta Medica)
13. Carter, M. E. (1980) Epidemiology. In Moll, J. M. H. (ed.) *Ankylosing Spondylitis*, pp. 16–25 (Edinburgh: Churchill Livingstone)
14. Ansell, B. M. (1978). Chronic arthritis in childhood. *Ann. Rheum. Dis.*, **37**, 107–20
15. Schaller, J. (1977) Ankylosing spondylitis of childhood onset. *Arthritis Rheum.*, **20** (Suppl.), 398–401
16. Masi, A. T. and Medsger, T. (1979). A new look at the epidemiology of ankylosing spondylitis and related syndromes. *Clin. Orthop. Related Res.*, **143**, 15–29
17. Arellano, J., Vallejo, M., Jimenez, J., Mintz, G. and Kretschmer, R. R. (1984). HLA-B27 and ankylosing spondylitis in Mexican Mestizo population. *Tissue Antigens*, **23**, 112–16
18. Ginsburg, W. W. and Cohen, M. D. (1983) Peripheral arthritis and ankylosing spondylitis: a review of 209 patients followed up for more than 20 years. *Mayo Clin. Proc.* **58**, 593–6
19. Lathinen, K. (1983). 76 patients with ankylosing spondylitis seen after 30 years of disease. *Scand. J. Rheumatol.*, **12**, 5–11
20. Dwosh, I. L., Resnick, D. and Becker, M. A. (1976) Hip involvement in ankylosing spondylitis. *Arthritis Rheum.*, **19**, 683–92

21. Riley, B. M., Ansell, B. M. and Bywaters, E. G. L. (1971) Radiological manifestations of ankylosing spondylitis according to age at onset. *Ann. Rheum. Dis.*,
**30,** 138–48

# 6

# MANAGEMENT OF ANKYLOSING SPONDYLITIS

*J. J. CALABRO*

## INTRODUCTION

The capriciousness of ankylosing spondylitis (AS) can create multiple and complex therapeutic problems. Consequently, a critical review of current forms of treatment seems timely. This report surveys and evaluates various therapeutic approaches, placing special emphasis on drug therapy and daily supportive measures.

Like most chronic rheumatic disorders, there is no cure for AS. Moreover, because the course of disease is so unpredictable, it is impossible to predict early what drugs or other forms of treatment may eventually be needed or what the ultimate prognosis may be. Nevertheless, considerable progress has been made in the management of AS so that much can be done for the young patient who is beginning to stoop as well as for the older patient already badly bent over with a 'poker spine'.

## COMPREHENSIVE MANAGEMENT

A programme of comprehensive management, clearly enhanced by early diagnosis and patient education, will contribute decisively to preventing or minimizing disability (Table 6.1). Such an improved outlook, however, requires several components of long-term care that include, first and foremost, the enthusiastic support of the patient

117

TABLE 6.1   Principles of comprehensive management in ankylosing spondylitis

---

1. Early diagnosis
2. Patient education and compliance
3. Direction and reassurance by a primary physician
4. Long-term care that includes:
   (a) Regular follow-up
   (b) Appropriate use of antirheumatic drugs
   (c) Supportive measures: daily exercises, postural training, night-time care, appropriate sports and recreation
   (d) Counselling: social, psychological, sexual, vocational, family, and genetic
   (e) Consultation, as needed, by a rheumatologist, ophthalmologist, orthopaedic surgeon, physiotherapist, or other
   (f) Participation in patient support groups, such as the Ankylosing Spondylitis Societies*

---

* For membership, patients may write to the following:
United States:   Ankylosing Spondylitis Association (ASA), 3985 Witzel Drive, Sherman Oaks, CA 91403, USA.
Great Britain:   The National Ankylosing Spondylitis Society (NASS), 6 Grosvenor Crescent, London SW1X 7ER, UK.
Canada:   The Arthritis Society, 920 Yonge Street, Toronto STE 420, Ontario, Canada M4 W3 17.

which, in turn, directly relates to the enthusiasm and efforts of the primary physician.

Goals of therapy

In the management of AS, the physician seeks to preserve an optimal lifestyle for the patient. The specific goals of therapy are threefold: (1) to prevent deformity and disability from progressive AS, (2) to recognize and control systemic (extra-articular) manifestations, and (3) to avoid undue hazards from various forms of treatment.

While these objectives can be achieved in the majority of patients, they are made possible only by comprehensive care that has both immediate and long-term objectives[1-14]. The physician must first relieve the patient's joint discomfort with anti-rheumatic drugs, then begin long-range planning to prevent, delay, or correct deformity. Consequently, daily exercises and other physical modalities are essential to maintain proper posture and range of motion.

## Patient education

The key to successful management is patient education. Pamphlets written for patients are available from a number of sources, including arthritis societies that have headquarters world-wide.

Management can succeed only with the active participation of the patient. To some patients, a drug regimen augmented by supportive measures such as daily exercises may appear too simple. Consequently, the physician must emphasize the excellent results obtainable by these seemingly undramatic measures. Moreover, the physician must explain that for the great majority of patients, medical measures alone will help them to maintain full and productive lives. Above all, patients should be educated about the nature of their disease and what they can reasonably expect from treatment. They should also be cautioned about therapeutic modalities they would be well advised to avoid, considering that Americans spend over a billion dollars yearly on arthritis quackery in their quest for quick and decisive cures.

Initially, of paramount importance are careful counselling and the planning of an individualized programme of management that the patient is able and willing to adopt as a way of life. This may help to motivate the reluctant patient as well as improve the cooperation of one only partially motivated. In long-term management, patients need continuous encouragement because they have the difficult task of adapting their lives to the disease. For the vast majority of patients, a good relationship with their physician is all the psychological support needed during prolonged management. At the outset, however, the physician should be alert to certain patients who may require the additional support of others, such as a vocational counsellor, social worker, or psychiatrist.

## NON-STEROIDAL ANTI-INFLAMMATORY DRUGS

Initial care begins with the appropriate use of non-steroidal anti-inflammatory drugs (NSAIDs) to suppress articular inflammation and discomfort. The drugs listed in Table 6.2 should be considered first, since these are of proven value in AS. Clearly, the task of selecting the most appropriate drug often rests more on tolerance or potential risks than on marginal differences in efficacy.[1,10,14].

TABLE 6.2  Chronologic listing of non-steroidal anti-inflammatory drugs in ankylosing spondylitis*

| Drug (US marketing) | Average daily dosage (range) for adults | Major adverse reactions |
|---|---|---|
| Acetylsalicylic acid† (1915) | 4 g (3–6 g) | Tinnitus, deafness, gastric distress, ulcer |
| Phenylbutazone‡ (1952) | 300 mg (100–400 mg) | Gastric distress, ulcer, stomatitis, nephrotoxicity, suppression of haematopoiesis§ |
| Indomethacin (1965) | 100 mg (25–100 mg) | Headache, drowsiness, gastric distress, ulcer |
| Naproxen (1976) | 750 mg (250–1000 mg) | Gastric distress, ulcer |
| Sulindac (1978) | 300 mg (100–400 mg) | Gastric distress, ulcer |
| Sustained-release indomethacin (1982) | 75 mg (75–150 mg) | Headache, drowsiness, gastric distress, ulcer · |

* Only non-steroidal anti-inflammatory drugs with United States Food and Drug Administration (FDA) approval for ankylosing spondylitis are included.
† Of those listed, only salicylates and naproxen have FDA approval for children under age 15  For children, the average daily dosage of acetylsalicylic acid is 80 mg/kg; the range is 60–110 mg/kg, and for naproxen 10–15 mg/kg.
‡ Currently recommended only after other drugs have been tried first  Oxyphenbutazone, marketed in 1961, is no longer available in most countries.
§ Including anaemia, leukopenia, agranulocytosis, thrombocytopenia, and aplastic anaemia

By suppressing axial and peripheral joint inflammation, pain, and stiffness, the NSAIDs facilitate exercise and other supportive measures that are the hallmark of treatment in AS[15]. While salicylates may be tried first, they are seldom adequate and in no way comparable to the effectiveness of either indomethacin or phenylbutazone. In fact, in a multicentred comparative trial of 49 patients with AS, in which each received 6 weeks of each of three drugs (acetylsalicylic acid, indomethacin, phenylbutazone), seven (only 15%) responded to acetylsalicylic acid in contrast to over 90% efficacy from either indomethacin or phenylbutazone[16].

## Salicylates

Acetylsalicylic acid is occasionally effective in AS, particularly when the patient has only minimal spinal discomfort. It may also be useful for AS patients with active disease confined to peripheral joints. However, acetylsalicylic acid is usually not effective when the shoulders or hips are involved or when there is moderate or severe spine involvement.

When used as an anti-inflammatory agent, the recommended initial dose of acetylsalicylic acid for adults is 3 g or more (Table 6.2). Since the amount needed to achieve anti-inflammatory effects varies widely from patient to patient, it may be wise to check serum salicylate levels, attaining therapeutic levels between 15 to 30 mg/dl. Moreover, the daily intake of salicylate should be increased slowly since it takes a week following each dosage change to attain a new steady-state serum level[17].

Ototoxicity is a common side-effect from the use of anti-inflammatory quantities of acetylsalicylic acid. In the event of tinnitus (ringing in the ears) or hearing loss, the drug should be stopped for 24 hours or until recovery of normal hearing and then resumed at a slightly lower dosage.

Toxic effects of acetylsalicylic acid include gastric irritation, occasionally with melena, and exacerbation of peptic ulcer. Salicylate preparations that are buffered with antacids may lessen symptoms of gastric irritation. This may also be accomplished by the use of enteric-coated tablets, although in some patients such coating interferes with gastrointestinal absorption.

Non-acetylated salicylates are also available[18]. Certain preparations, such as salicylsalicylic acid (salsalate), bypass the stomach and dissolve in the alkaline medium of the small intestine. Moreover, salicylsalicylic acid inhibits cyclo-oxygenase only one-fifth as much as acetylsalicylic acid[19]. Consequently, there is minimal gastrointestinal irritation, bleeding, and ulceration due to salsalate. Many non-acetylated salicylates do not inhibit platelet aggregation or prolong the bleeding time, and can be administered twice daily.

## Phenylbutazone

In patients with moderate or severe pain and stiffness of the spine, hips or shoulders, phenylbutazone will prove to be more satisfactory than salicylates. Most patients initially require 100 mg of phenyl-butazone administered three or four times daily, while patients with minimal disease activity may need only a single 100-mg tablet either on arising or at bedtime (Table 6.2). On the basis of a retrospective study, it has been reported that phenylbutazone may alter favourably the natural course of AS[20]. Continuous treatment with the drug con-trolled or inhibited syndesmophyte formation and ossification of para-spinal ligaments.

Common adverse reactions to phenylbutazone include epigastric distress, nausea, and vomiting. Pre-existing peptic ulcer may be aggra-vated; occasionally, massive bleeding or even perforation may occur. Other side-effects include oedema from retention of sodium and chlor-ide, stomatitis, hepatitis, and a pruritic maculopapular skin eruption. Because of drug interaction, when phenylbutazone is used con-comitantly with anticoagulants, the prothrombin time must be checked regularly to prevent bleeding[21,22].

Signs of nephrotoxicity with haematuria, or bone marrow sup-pression manifest by anaemia, leukopenia, agranulocytosis, throm-bocytopenia, or aplastic anaemia, are rare. Nevertheless, a complete blood count, platelet count, and urinalysis must be performed weekly for the initial two months of drug therapy and monthly thereafter. The occurrence of sore throat, fever, or rash during treatment with phenylbutazone should alert the physician to the possibility of agran-ulocytosis and should lead to immediate cessation of the drug[2]. Agran-ulocytosis occurs primarily in younger patients, often after a few days or weeks of therapy with phenylbutazone, and is readily reversible when the drug is discontinued. On the other hand, aplastic anaemia occurs more frequently in the elderly, is more apt to evolve insidiously after prolonged drug therapy, and is more likely to prove fatal.

## Indomethacin

One of the earliest reports of indomethacin in AS dates back to 1968[23]. It detailed a five-year clinical trial of the drug in 28 patients. As judged by several criteria, including articular pain, duration of morning stiffness, onset of fatigue, and joint mobility, the overall response of indomethacin was rated as good in 21 patients, fair in five, and poor in two. After receiving indomethacin for an average of 33 months, 21 of the 28 patients were classified in the American Rheumatism Association functional class I[24]. Only one patient had been so classified prior to the drug trial. The average Westergren erythrocyte sedimentation rate for all 28 patients decreased during the drug trial from 39 to 26 mm/h ($p < 0.01$, Student's $t$ test). Consequently, the results of this long-term trial demonstrate that indomethacin alters favourably the course of AS.

Central nervous system toxicity, particularly headache and drowsiness, and gastrointestinal side-effects, frequently transient and generally tolerated upon reduction of the daily dosage, occurred most often with a daily administration of 200 mg of indomethacin[23]. In fact, four of the eight patients who experienced adverse reactions were taking 200 mg of the drug daily. Indomethacin was withdrawn from three patients, two because of a poor response to the drug, and one because of an adverse reaction.

In 1981, 18 years after the first patients were entered into this trial, it was possible to locate and reassess 14 patients[5,15]. Of the 14, four had achieved remission and required no further drug therapy. Indomethacin had been withdrawn in four patients, two because of gastrointestinal side-effects and two because of a more favourable effect from another NSAID. The remaining six patients continue to receive indomethacin at an average daily dosage of 100 mg (range, 75–100 mg) and continue to benefit from its long-term use.

The initial dose of indomethacin is 25 mg given two or three times daily. The daily dosage can be increased by 25 mg at about weekly intervals until a satisfactory response is obtained or the daily maximum of 200 mg is reached (Table 6.2). Most patients require 100 mg daily. However, some patients may need only a single 25-mg capsule on arising, whereas others with severe back or hip involvement may require as much as 200 mg daily. To avoid gastric upset, patients should be advised to take their capsules with meals or at bedtime with milk or food.

One disadvantage with the use of the 25- and 50-mg indomethacin capsules is the need to administer each of these preparations three or four times daily. Alternatively, the newer 75-mg sustained-release form can be given once or twice daily. Consequently, it may be a more convenient way of prescribing indomethacin, especially suited for patients who tend to be non-compliant[25]. Indomethacin suppositories of 50 or 100 mg are also available and can be administered at bedtime to allay night time discomfort as well as early morning stiffness.

## Naproxen and sulindac

Naproxen[26,27] and sulindac[28-30] are additional drugs with proven efficacy in AS. Because of their longer half-life, 13 hours for naproxen and 16 hours for sulindac, each can be given twice daily and are therefore aptly suited for patients who tend to be non-compliant. The daily maximum should not exceed 1000 mg for naproxen and 400 mg for sulindac (Table 6.2).

A number of other NSAIDs are also effective in AS[7,10,31-36]. Moreover, additional ones are on the horizon, and some may be approved and released for use shortly after this report has been published. Regardless of the choice, patients should be monitored and warned of potential adverse reactions. Finally, every effort should be made to reduce the daily dose to the lowest one possible. Drug withdrawal should be attempted slowly and only after active articular disease has been suppressed for at least several months.

## Adverse reactions and contraindications

The NSAIDs share a common core of side-effects (Table 6.3). They differ widely, however, in their innate propensity for inducing these. For example, ototoxicity is more apt to occur with salicylates, central nervous system toxicity with indomethacin and sulindac, sodium and fluid retention with phenylbutazone, while palpitations and pneumonitis are more frequent with naproxen. Except for phenylbutazone, fatal aplastic anaemia is rarely observed with NSAID therapy.

Although phenylbutazone and acetylsalicylic acid influence the

TABLE 6.3   Adverse reactions common to all non-steroidal anti-inflammatory drugs

---

1. Gastrointestinal upset: nausea, vomiting, dyspepsia, diarrhoea, constipation, melena
2. Major gastrointestinal bleeding, ulcer, or perforation
3. Toxic hepatitis
4. Mucocutaneous: skin rash, pruritus, urticaria, alopecia, stomatitis
5. Ocular toxicity: reversible blurring of vision
6. Ototoxicity: reversible ringing in ears and difficulty with hearing
7. Central nervous system toxicity: headache, drowsiness, dizziness, confusion, lightheadedness, agitation, lethargy, malaise, depression
8. Cardiopulmonary toxicity: palpitations, arrhythmias, pneumonitis; leg oedema and congestive heart failure from sodium and fluid retention
9. Haematological: alteration of platelet function, prolongation of the bleeding time, aplastic anaemia (rare)
10. Nephrotoxicity, including the nephrotic syndrome

---

hypoprothrombinaemia produced by anticoagulants, most other NSAIDs do not. Nevertheless, when any NSAID is prescribed along with anticoagulant therapy, the patient should be carefully observed for alterations of the prothrombin time.

The NSAIDs are contraindicated in patients with the syndrome of bronchospasm, nasal polyps, and angioedema precipitated by acetylsalicylic acid or other NSAIDs. In the United States, except for salicylates, naproxen and tolmetin sodium, safe conditions for use in children under 15 years of age have not been established. Nor have safe conditions for their prescribing in pregnant and nursing women been established[37,38]. All NSAIDs mask the usual signs and symptoms of infection. All should be used with special care in the elderly[39,40].

## OTHER ANTIRHEUMATIC THERAPY

Additional forms of antirheumatic therapy may or may not benefit patients with AS[1,7]. These are listed in Table 6.4, along with their current status.

### Analgesics

Drugs that are primarily analgesic, i.e. reduce pain but have no anti-inflammatory effect, are often used in AS. These include drugs like acetaminophen and propoxyphene as well as narcotics. However, these drugs lack the anti-inflammatory property essential for suppression of inflammation in the peripheral joints or spine of patients with active AS. This is also true of muscle relaxants. Consequently, muscle relaxants, like analgesics, can be prescribed for short periods as additional

TABLE 6.4   Current status of antirheumatic therapy other than the non-steroidal anti-inflammatory drugs in ankylosing spondylitis

| Therapy | Current status |
| --- | --- |
| Analgesics, muscle relaxants | Adjunctively for short term, but not as basic drugs |
| Irradiation of the spine | Not routinely recommended |
| Remittive agents | Of no benefit, except for levamisole (usefulness limited by toxicity) and sulphasalazine |
| Oral adrenocorticosteroids | Of limited value |
| IV methylprednisolone pulse therapy | Promising but needs further evaluation |
| Topical corticosteroids | Effective for acute anterior uveitis |
| Intra-articular steroids | Beneficial for one or two active peripheral joints |

drugs for severe pain and spasm. They should never be used, however, as basic drugs in management.

The local application of heat or cold is also helpful in reducing pain, thereby facilitating exercise. Moreover, early-morning stiffness and spine discomfort can be effectively reduced by either a warm tub bath or shower. Biofeedback training is another approach to relieving muscle tension and pain. Other physical modalities to reduce pain include diathermy, ultrasound, and transcutaneous electrical nerve stimulation (TENS).

Irradiation of the spine

This older form of therapy for AS is no longer in vogue, now that the NSAIDs are available. However, before the discovery of phenylbutazone, the first NSAID (Table 6.2), irradiation to the spine was commonly used in the management of AS.

This approach has justifiably come into disrepute as a routine form of AS therapy. Radiotherapy renders AS patients twice as susceptible to acute myelogenous leukaemia as the general population[41]. The risk of leukaemia rises sharply as the mean dose to spinal marrow reaches 500 r. Moreover, in a 1965 survey of more than 14 500 AS patients who had received radiotherapy at some time between 1935 and 1954, 49 had died from acute myelogenous leukaemia six to eight, and even as long as 15, years following radiotherapy[41]. Other complications from spine irradiation include aplastic anaemia and cancer in general[41], as well as basal cell carcinoma[42]. It is important, therefore, to examine previous radiation sites carefully since cutaneous neoplasia of the spine may develop up to 50 years later[42].

## Remittive agents

Although beneficial in rheumatoid arthritis, the remittive (slow-acting) agents, such as oral or intramuscular gold, the antimalarial drugs, d-penicillamine, and azathioprine appear to be of no benefit in AS[1,7,43]. However, except for d-penicillamine, there have been no formal trials of these agents in AS. In a recent trial of d-penicillamine, there was no difference between placebo and active drug in 20 patients evaluated for six months[43].

Based on a double-blind, placebo-controlled study of 12 weeks, levamisole proved to be effective in AS[44]. Currently, however, because of major toxicity, the drug cannot be recommended for routine use in AS[7]. Sulfasalazine, a highly effective drug for ulcerative colitis and regional enteritis[45], has been tried recently in AS[46,47]. Preliminary results are promising, including those of a double-blind trial in which sulfasalazine was compared to placebo in 37 patients[46]. The dosage of sulfasalazine is built up slowly to between 2 and 4 g daily and a favourable response may occur anywhere from a few months to a full year of drug therapy.

## Adrenocorticosteroids

ACTH and oral adrenocorticosteroids have limited therapeutic value in long-term management because of their potential for serious toxicity[7]. In fact, their long-term use may be risky, predisposing patients to steroid-induced compression fractures of the spine and ischaemic necrosis of the femoral head. Of the many good reasons not to promote prolonged steroid therapy, most cogent are the results of earlier comparative trials in which better efficacy was achieved with either indomethacin or phenylbutazone[6].

The role of adrenocorticosteroids in AS was revived in 1981 following a report on the use of 1 g pulses of intravenous methylprednisolone in patients failing to respond to NSAIDs[48]. In this open study, there was a dramatic response lasting for up to 14 months, depending of the number of methylprednisolone pulses given. This favourable response has been confirmed in a more recent open study of eight patients, but the improvement in pain, stiffness, and spinal movement lasted for only one or two months[7]. Improvement was paralleled by a fall in acute phase reactants[49]. A double-blind, placebo-controlled trial of methylprednisolone pulse therapy in AS is currently being conducted[7]. Clearly, the use of this form of therapy both for acute exacerbations and in prolonged treatment needs further evaluation.

For therapy of acute anterior uveitis, topical corticosteroids (and mydriatics) are usually satisfactory so that oral corticosteroids are rarely required. The use of intra-articular steroids may also be beneficial, particularly when one or two peripheral joints are more severely inflamed than others, thereby compromising rehabilitation, exercise, and other supportive measures[6].

## SUPPORTIVE MEASURES

Restoring joint function or correcting deformity is much more difficult than preventing it. Yet, even advanced deformities of the spine or marked limitation of the chest cage will often yield readily to a programme of exercise (Figure 6.1). The objective of all supportive measures, whether they be postural training, therapeutic exercise, or recreational therapy, is to build up muscle groups that oppose the direction of potential deformity and thus to strengthen extensor rather than flexor muscle groups. Moreover, a host of specialists may be needed for long-term care (Table 6.5). Finally, regardless of the course

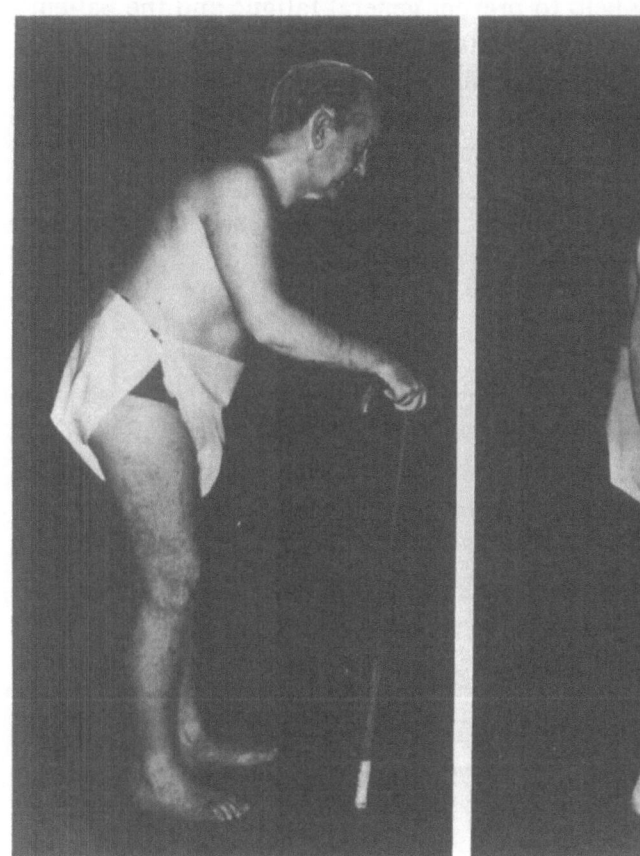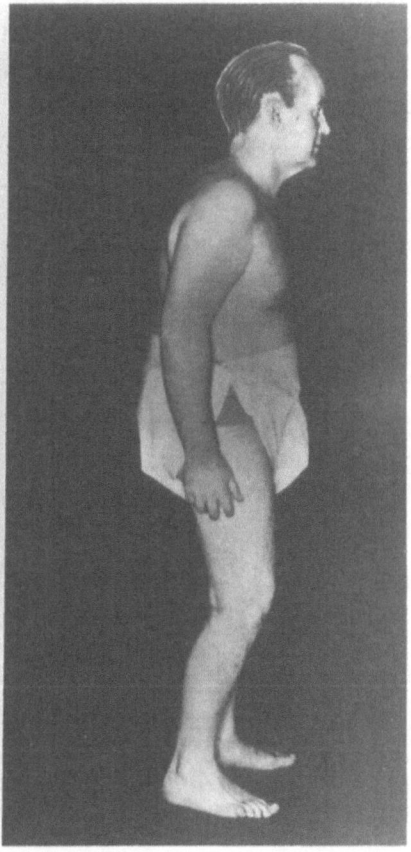

FIGURE 6.1   *Left:* The patient is barely able to see ahead because of pronounced flexion deformity of the spine; *right:* after two months of daily extension exercises, however, the patient is almost upright again.

of disease, the psychosocial and rehabilitative needs of the patient deserve careful attention in long-range planning.

## Rest and activity

A proper balance between rest and activity must be provided for each patient. Prolonged bed rest promotes vertebral osteoporosis and should therefore be avoided. For most patients seven or eight hours of sleep at night is sufficient. When needed, however, short rest periods

129

during the day may help to prevent general fatigue and the patient's tendency to 'droop' in the late afternoon.

The amount of daily rest will depend on the degree of disease activity. Some restrictions may be necessary when the patient has severe fatigue or when the disease flares and becomes more active than usual. Even then, however, the patient should be encouraged to continue daily exercise. Above all, the patient must stay active in order to keep the spine as mobile as possible.

## Postural training

To prevent the automatic tendency to stoop since it helps to alleviate spinal pain, the patient must always consciously stand as erect as possible and to walk 'tall'. Even when picking up objects from the floor, the patient should not bend over but squat, keeping the back upright. The patient must always sit erect, preferably on a chair with

TABLE 6.5   Consultations for special problems in ankylosing spondylitis

| Special problem | Referral to |
| --- | --- |
| Refractory spondylitis* | Rheumatologist |
| Reversible spine/joint limitation | Physiotherapist |
| Heel involvement† | Rheumatologist/orthopaedic surgeon/podiatrist |
| Fixed deformity | Orthopaedic surgeon |
| Vertebral fracture, subluxation | Orthopaedic surgeon/neurosurgeon |
| Acute anterior uveitis | Ophthalmologist |
| Cauda equina syndrome | Neurologist/urologist |
| Aortic insufficiency‡ | Cardiologist |
| Pulmonary fibrosis | Pulmonary specialist |
| Pulmonary aspergillosis | Pulmonary specialist |
| Drug-induced GI problems | Gastroenterologist |
| Obesity | Nutritionist |
| Psychological problems | Psychiatrist/psychologist |

* Unresponsive to a succession of NSAIDs at maximum dosages.
† Including plantar fasciitis and achillotendinitis or achillobursitis from ankylosing spondylitis.
‡ As well as for other cardiac problems associated with ankylosing spondylitis, such as symptomatic heart block or pericarditis.

a hard, straight back and seat. Although suitable braces may help to maintain good posture, most patients do well without them.

## Night-time care

Night-time is often forgotten in the overall management of arthritis. Patients not only need adequate hours of rest at night, but they must sleep on a firm mattress supported by a rigid board. Consequently, unless firmly constructed, water beds are to be avoided. Moreover, no pillows are to be used under the hips or knees and only a small one, if any, under the neck.

## Therapeutic exercise

Prescribed by a physician or a qualified associate, exercise must become an intrinsic part of the patient's daily life. Therapeutic exercise must be tailored not only to the degree of spine involvement, but also the patient's age, strength, and capacity to cooperate. Moreover, exercises must be performed daily and reevaluated periodically as part of the patient's regular follow-up.

Spine extension and chest-cage stretching are the most important exercises and may be done either standing or lying down.

### Spine extension exercise

Lying on the abdomen, the patient stretches the arms out at shoulder level, then raises the head, chest, shoulders, and arms off the bed as far as possible. The patient then relaxes and repeats the exercise 10 to 20 times.

### Chest cage expansion

Lying on the back, the patient clasps the hands behind the head. The patient then pulls the elbows to the bed while breathing in deeply, holds the breath in for a count of 10, exhales, and relaxes. The exercise should be repeated 10 to 20 times.

131

*Combined exercise for spine extension and chest expansion*

Because of its dual objectives, this is an extremely useful exercise (Figure 6.2). The exercise is repeated 10 to 20 times and, depending on the need, is performed once, twice, or three times daily.

Specific exercises may also be provided to improve the function of

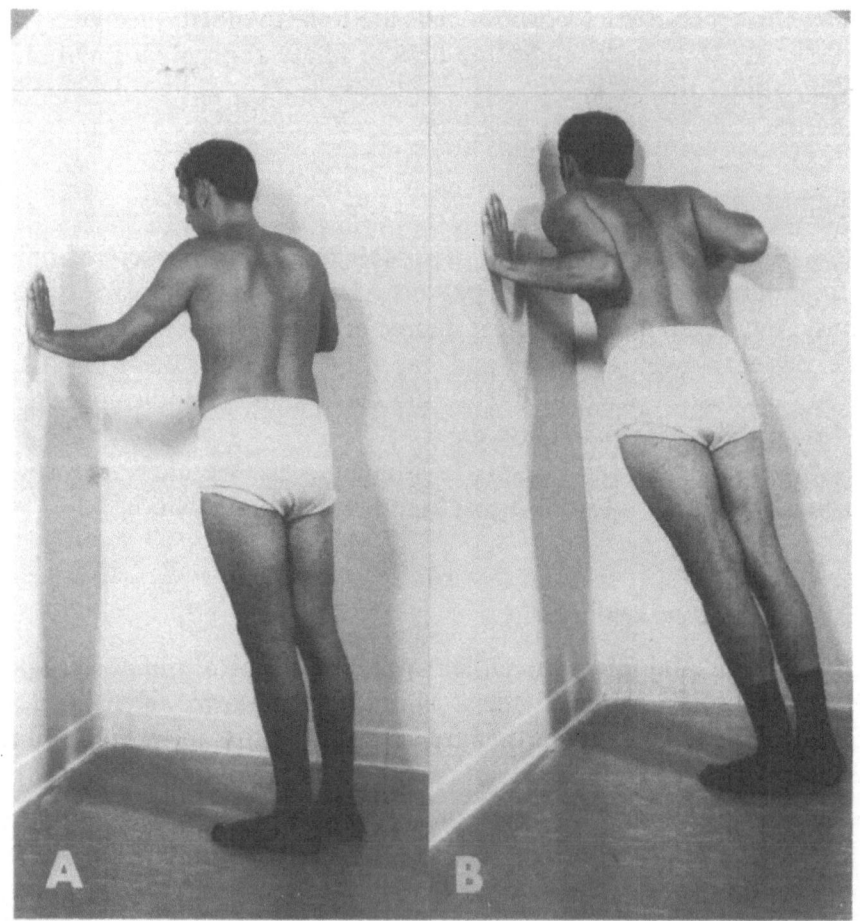

FIGURE 6.2 For an exercise that combines spinal extension and chest expansion: (A) patient faces corner while touching opposite walls at shoulder height; (B) patient bends elbows and leans forward while extending neck (looking up) and breathing in as deeply as possible.

132

hips, shoulders, or other involved peripheral joints. When indicated, exercises that stretch calf and hamstring muscles should also be included[50].

## Hamstring stretching

While lying on the floor with knees bent, the patient brings one leg up toward the chest, then grasps the back of the thigh with the hands, straightening the leg at the knee as much as possible. With toes bent down toward the knee, the patient slowly pulls the thigh forward keeping the knee as straight as possible. The patient holds the position for a five-second count, relaxes to the starting position, and repeats the exercise with the other leg. Hamstring stretching should be performed five times with each leg.

## Recreational therapy

Kinesiological analyses of various sports and recreation have determined which are therapeutically useful[51]. For example, swimming, archery, racquet-type games, and most forms of dancing appear to be suitable for patients, whereas bowling, golfing, and jogging are usually inappropriate.

Swimming encourages motion of the chest cage, spine, shoulders, and hips. The wedge kick is particularly effective in promoting hip movement. If shoulder motion is limited, the back stroke must be avoided, but the side stroke or a modified breast stroke may be used.

Archery aids motion of the chest cage, spine, and shoulders, as do racquet sports, such as badminton and tennis. Games like dart-throwing promote extension and rotation of the spine, shoulder, and hip as well as deep breathing.

Dancing enhances both spine extension and chest expansion. This is true of most forms of ballroom dancing, such as the fox-trot, waltz, rumba, and swing. Some forms of dancing, such as the twist, the bump, the hustle, and disco dancing, should be avoided, however, because they require abrupt and extensive twisting motion that may aggravate the spine.

Bowling is contraindicated for patients with marked restrictions of spine, shoulder, or hip movement. Jogging or long periods of golf-putting promote forceful flexion of the spine that may be harmful. The use of a long putter or restricting golf practice to the driving range is a practical alternative. Surf-casting may be difficult for individuals with marked limitation of the spine or hips. On the other hand, bait-casting, fly-casting, or trolling are encouraged, since they require less physical strain.

In general, sports and activities that encourage an upright posture and spinal extension are recommended. Even activities like golf, billiards, bowling, and bicycling, which may encourage a forward stooped posture, need not be avoided if compensations are made (e.g. shorter golf swing, lighter bowling ball, high handlebars).

A case in point of recreational activity inappropriate for AS is provided by a 26-year-old man who rapidly developed a fixed lumbar kyphosis from ten-speed bicycling[52]. His deformity resulted from riding flexed forward on a ten-speed bicycle for several hours daily while his spondylitis was active. This case serves to demonstrate that exercise, whether formal or recreational, must be geared to promote extension rather than flexion, thereby opposing the direction of potential deformity.

### Gymnasium and aerobic exercises

Because of the current popularity of health clubs, some caution on the use of gym equipment is appropriate. Machines that emphasize arm and leg conditioning are recommended. Equipment for toning up muscles and promoting spinal extension can be helpful, but machines that put undue strain on the back and neck should be avoided.

Aerobic exercising is recommended for all patients with AS. Because of disease limitations, however, some patients may need modified programmes of aerobic exercise (e.g. use of a stationary bicycle, exercising in a hot tub). Also, modified forms of yoga may be valuable because of its breathing and stretching effects[50].

### Sexual activity

AS can severely sap sexual activity and pleasure. Consequently, patients should discuss openly and freely any sexual problems induced by their disease[53,54].

Most forms of sexual intercourse are possible for both men and women, even in the presence of flexion deformities of the spine. Men with spondylitis are often reluctant to have intercourse in the top position, because spinal flexion causes back pain and spasm. In this situation, the supine position, in which the man lies flat on his back, may be more comfortable. On the other hand, intercourse with the patient lying on the side might be more suitable for patients with severe deformity of the back or hip.

## Nutrition

Apart from the promise of dietary studies currently being investigated in England, there is no special diet for AS. In fact, no specific food has anything to do with causing AS and no specific diet will cure it. Consequently, advise patients that what they may hear or see advertised to the contrary has no scientific validity.

The ideal diet for AS is a well-balanced and nourishing one because proper nutrition is essential for good health whether you have AS or not. Sometimes AS can make a patient run down and underweight, leading to fatigue and lowered resistance. These patients will need extra nourishment, over and above a normal and well-balanced diet. On the other hand, overweight patients need a reduction diet that is monitored by a physician or nutritionist. Otherwise, obesity puts enormous pressure on the spine; as the belly thrusts out, the buttocks push back to offset the extra weight in front and the normal curvature of the spine deepens abnormally. Obesity not only places extra burden on the spine but it also adversely affects weight-bearing joints, such as the hips and knees.

## SURGICAL INTERVENTION

Reconstructive surgery should be contemplated only after all conservative measures have failed. For patients with advanced deformities, whether of the spine, hips, or other joints, surgical corrections is now feasible[55-64]. This requires, however, a very careful assessment, meticulous preoperative planning, and precise attention to operative and anaesthesia techniques to assure consistent success without major risk to the patient.[57,65,66].

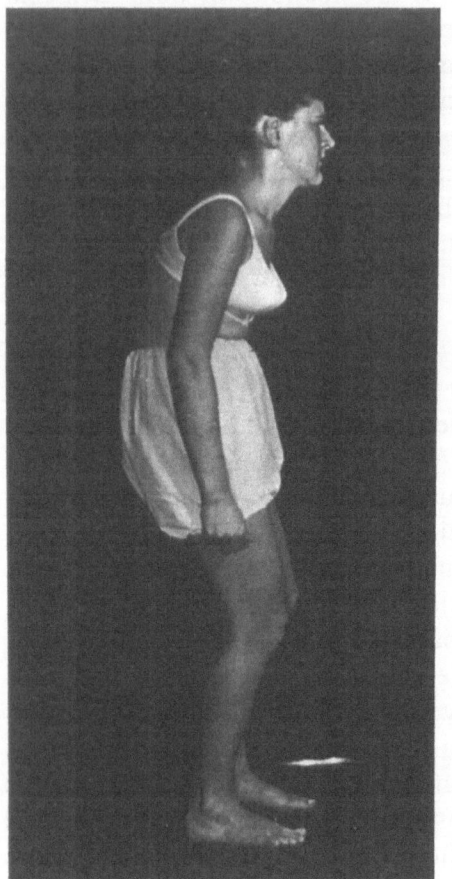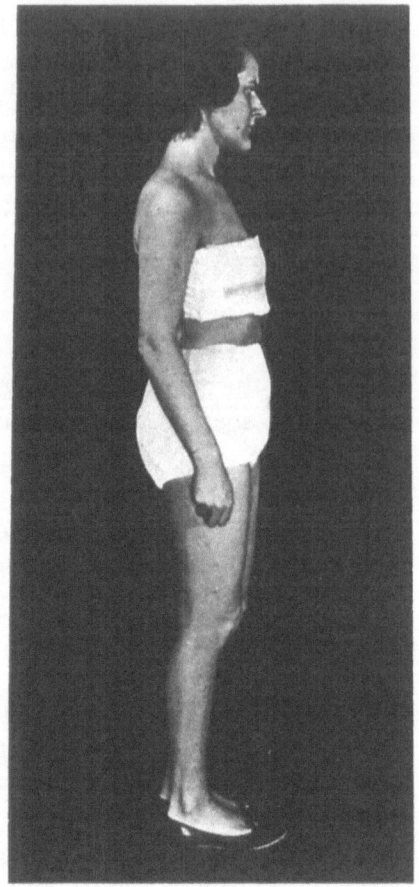

FIGURE 6.3 (*left*) Six months of therapeutic exercises did not alter the stooped posture of a 26-year-old woman. (*right*) Surgery produced dramatic improvement in this patient, shown one year after lumbar wedge osteotomy.

While the technique of lumbar osteotomy is constantly improving, it is still an extensive and delicate procedure that also requires prolonged postoperative care (Figure 6.3)[6,55–62]. Total hip replacement may also provide dramatic results initially, but the subsequent development of bony ankylosis above the prosthesis may result in failure[63,64]. While spine, hip, or other reconstructive measures are a last resort, correction of vertebral fracture or dislocation are urgent problems because of their potential for nerve root injury or compression of the spinal cord[6].

## References

1. Calabro, J.J. (1985). Drug therapy of juvenile rheumatoid arthritis and the seronegative spondyloarthropathies. In Roth, S. H. (ed.) *Drug Therapy in Rheumatology*, pp. 115–80. (Littleton, MA: PSG)
2. Khan, M. A. (1984). Ankylosing spondylitis. In Calin, A. (ed.) *Spondyloarthropathies*, pp. 69–117. (Orlando, FL: Grune and Stratton)
3. Calin, A. (1985). Ankylosing spondylitis. *Clin. Rheum. Dis.*, **11**, 41–60
4. Calin, A. and Fries, J. F. (1978). *Ankylosing Spondylitis: Discussions in Patient Management*. (Garden City, NY: Medical Examination Publishing)
5. Calabro, J.J. (1985). Sustained-release indomethacin in the management of ankylosing spondylitis. *Am. J. Med.*, **79** (Suppl. 4C), 39–51
6. Calabro, J.J. (1968). An appraisal of the medical and surgical management of ankylosing spondylitis. *Clin. Orthop.*, **60**, 125–48
7. Richter, M. B. (1985). Management of the seronegative spondyloarthropathies. *Clin. Rheum. Dis.*, **11**, 147–69
8. Calabro, J.J. (1986). The seronegative spondyloarthropathies. A graduated approach to management. *Postgrad. Med.*, **80**, 173–88
9. Calabro, J.J. and Maltz, B. A. (1970). Ankylosing spondylitis. *N. Engl. J. Med.*, **282**, 606–10
10. Hill, A. G. S. (1980). Drug therapy. In Moll, J. M. H. (ed.) *Ankylosing Spondylitis*, pp. 163–75. (Edinburgh: Churchill Livingstone)
11. Wynn Parry, C. B. and Deary, J. (1980). Physical measures in rehabilitation. In Moll, J. M. H. (ed.) *Ankylosing Spondylitis*, pp. 214–26. (Edinburgh: Churchill Livingstone)
12. Chamberlain, M. A. (1980). Socio-domestic and psychological factors in management. In Moll, J. M. H. (ed.) *Ankylosing Spondylitis*, pp. 227–35. (Edinburgh: Churchill Livingstone)
13. Anderson, J. A. D. (1980). Occupational factors in management. In Moll, J. M. H. (ed.) *Ankylosing Spondylitis*, pp. 236–42. (Edinburgh: Churchill Livingstone)
14. Calabro, J.J., Eyvazzadeh, C. and Weber, C. A. (1986). Contemporary management of ankylosing spondylitis. *Compr. Ther.*, **12**, 11–18
15. Calabro, J.J. (1982). Appraisal of efficacy and tolerability of INDOCIN[R] (indomethacin, MSD) in acute gout and moderate to severe ankylosing spondylitis. *Semin. Arthritis Rheum.*, **12** (Suppl. 1), 112–16
16. Godfrey, R. G., Calabro, J.J., Mills, D. and Maltz, B. A. (1972). A double-blind crossover trial of aspirin, indomethacin and phenylbutazone in ankylosing spondylitis. *Arthritis Rheum.*, **15**, 110 (Abst)
17. Dromgoole, S. H., Furst, D. E. and Paulus, H. E. (1981). Rational approaches to the use of salicylates in the treatment of rheumatoid arthritis. *Semin. Arthritis Rheum.*, **11**, 257–83
18. Roth, S. H. (1980). Salicylates: Revolution versus evolution. In Roth, S. H. (ed.) *New Directions in Arthritis Therapy*, pp. 23–36. (Littleton, MA: PSG)
19. Calabro, J.J., Eyvazzadeh, C. and Weber, C. (1986). Juvenile rheumatoid arthritis (Letter). *N. Engl. J. Med.*, **315**, 1096

20. Boersma, J. W. (1976). Retardation of ossification of the lumbar vertebral column in ankylosing spondylitis by means of phenylbutazone. *Scand. J. Rheumatol.*, **5**, 60–4
21. Eisen, M. J. (1964). Combined effect of sodium warfarin and phenylbutazone. *J. Am. Med. Assoc.*, **189**, 64–5
22. Fox, S. L. (1964). Potentiation of anticoagulants caused by pyrazole compounds. *J. Am. Med. Assoc.*, **188**, 320–1
23. Calabro, J. J. and Amante, C. M. (1968). Indomethacin in ankylosing spondylitis. *Arthritis Rheum.*, **11**, 56–64
24. Steinbrocker, O., Traeger, C. H. and Batterman, R. C. (1949). Therapeutic criteria in rheumatoid arthritis. *J. Am. Med. Assoc.*, **140**, 659–62
25. Katz, W. A. (1982). Compliance. *Semin. Arthritis Rheum.*, **12** (Suppl. 1), 132–5
26. Ansell, B. M., Major, G., Liyanage, S. P., Gumpel, J. M., Seifert, M. H., Mathews, J. A. and Engler, C. (1978). A comparative study of Butacote and Naprosyn in ankylosing spondylitis. *Ann. Rheum. Dis.*, **37**, 436–9
27. Segre, E. J. (1979). Naproxen. *Clin. Rheum. Dis.*, **5**, 411–26
28. Liebling, M. R., Altman, R. D., Benedek, T. G., Bennahum, D. A., Blaschke, J. A., Bower, R. J., Calabro, J. J., Caldwell, J. R., Collins, R. L., Felt, J., Hamaty, D., Jimeneo, C. V., Umbenhauer, E. R. and Willkens, R. F. (1975). A double-blind, multiclinic trial of sulindac (MK-231) in the treatment of ankylosing spondylitis. *Arthritis Rheum.*, **18**, 411 (Abst)
29. Rhymer, A. R. (1979). Sulindac. *Clin. Rheum. Dis.*, **5**, 553–68
30. Gibson, T. and Laurent, R. (1980). Sulindac and indomethacin in the treatment of ankylosing spondylitis: A double-blind cross-over study. *Rheumatol. Rehabil.*, **19**, 189–92
31. Calin, A. (1983). Clinical use of tolmetin sodium in patients with ankylosing spondylitis: A review. *J. Clin. Pharmacol.*, **23**, 301–8
32. Lomen, P. L., Turner, L. F., Lamborn, K. R. and Brinn, E. L. (1986). Flurbiprofen in the treatment of ankylosing spondylitis. A comparison with indomethacin. *Am. J. Med.*, **80** (Suppl. 3A), 127–32
33. Lomen, P. L., Turner, L. F., Lamborn, K. R., Brinn, E. L. and Sattler, L. P. (1986). Flurbiprofen in the treatment of ankylosing spondylitis. A comparison with phenylbutazone. *Am. J. Med.*, **80** (Suppl. 3A), 120–6
34. Calabro, J. J. (1986). Efficacy of diclofenac in ankylosing spondylitis. *Am. J. Med.*, **80** (Suppl. 4B), 58–63
35. Nahir, A. M. and Scharf, Y. (1980). A comparative study of diclofenac and sulindac in ankylosing spondylitis. *Rheumatol. Rehabil.*, **19**, 193–8
36. Franssen, M. J. A. M., van de Putte, L. B. A. and Gribnau, F. W. J. (1985). IgA serum levels and disease activity in ankylosing spondylitis: a prospective study. *Ann. Rheum. Dis.*, **44**, 766–71
37. Needs, C. J. and Brooks, P. M. (1985). Antirheumatic medication in pregnancy. *Br. J. Rheumatol.*, **24**, 282–90
38. Needs, C. J. and Brooks, P. M. (1985). Antirheumatic medication during lactation. *Br. J. Rheumatol.*, **24**, 291–7
39. Calabro, J. J. (1985). Analgesic and anti-inflammatory therapy in the elderly. *Am. J. Med.*, **79** (Suppl. 4B), 33–4
40. Ouslander, J. G. (1981). Drug therapy in the elderly. *Ann Intern. Med.*, **95**, 711–22
41. Court-Brown, W. M. and Doll, R. (1957). Mortality from cancer and other causes after radiotherapy for ankylosing spondylitis. *Am. J. Med.*, **22**, 580–92

42. Good, A. E., Diaz, L. A. and Bowerman, R. A. (1980). Basal cell carcinomas following roentgen therapy of ankylosing spondylitis. *Arthritis Rheum.*, **23,** 1065–7

43. Steven, M. M., Morrison, M. and Sturrock, R. D. (1985). Penicillamine in ankylosing spondylitis: A double-blind placebo controlled trial. *J. Rheumatol.*, **12,** 735–7

44. Goebel, K. M., Schubotz, R., Goebel, F. D., Hahn, E. and Neurath, F. (1977). Levamisole-induced immunostimulation in spondylarthropathies. *Lancet*, **2,** 214–17

45. Peppercorn, M. A. (1984). Sulfasalazine: Pharmacology, clinical use, toxicity, and related new drug development. *Ann. Intern. Med.*, **101,** 377–86

46. Feltelius, N. and Hallgren, R. (1986). Sulphasalazine in ankylosing spondylitis. *Ann. Rheum. Dis.*, **45,** 396–9

47. Mielants, H., Veys, E. M. and Joos, R. (1986). Sulphasalazine (Salazopyrin) in the treatment of enterogenic reactive synovitis and ankylosing spondylitis with peripheral arthritis. *Clin. Rheumatol.*, **5,** 80–3

48. Mintz, G., Enriquez, R. D., Mercado, U., Robles, E. J., Jimenez, F. J. and Gutierrez G. (1981). Intravenous methylprednisolone pulse therapy in severe ankylosing spondylitis. *Arthritis Rheum.*, **5,** 734–6

49. Richter, M. B., Woo, P. and Panayi, G. S. (1983). The effects of intravenous pulse methylprednisolone on immunological and inflammatory processes in ankylosing spondylitis. *Clin. Exp. Immunol.*, **53,** 51–9

50. Ostrow, S. and Rosenberg, M. (1985). Maintaining good posture and flexibility. In R. L. Swezey (ed.) *Straight Talk on Ankylosing Spondylitis*, pp. 9–26. (Sherman Oaks, CA: Ankylosing Spondylitis Association, Inc.)

51. Edwards, M. H., Calabro, J. J., Avedon, E. M., Arje, F. B. and Berryman, D. L. (1966). Therapeutic recreation for the patient with ankylosing spondylitis. *Arch. Phys. Med. Rehabil.*, **47,** 77–83

52. Taylor, P. W. (1980). Ankylosing spondylitis with unusual spinal deformity: A case report. *J. Rheumatol.*, **7,** 919–22

53. Elst, P., Sybesma, T., van der Stadt, R. J., Prins, A. P. A., Hissink Muller, W. and den Butter, A. (1984). Sexual problems in rheumatoid arthritis and ankylosing spondylitis. *Arthritis Rheum.*, **27,** 217–20

54. Zant, J. L., Dekker-Saeys, A. J., van den Burgh, I. C., Kolman, A. and van der Stadt, R. J. (1982). Asthenia, ambition and educational level in patients suffering from ankylosing spondylitis: a controlled study of personality features as compared to rheumatoid arthritis and unspecified low back pain. *Clin. Rheumatol.*, **4,** 243–50

55. Simmons, E. H. (1977). Kyphotic deformity of spine in ankylosing spondylitis. *Clin. Orthop.*, **128,** 65–77

56. Law, W. A. (1976). Ankylosing spondylitis and spinal osteotomy. *Proc. R. Soc. Med.*, **69,** 715–20

57. McMaster, M. J. and Coventry, M. B. (1973). Spinal osteotomy in ankylosing spondylitis. Techniques, complications, and long-term results. *Mayo Clin. Proc.*, **48,** 476–86

58. Scudese, V. A. and Calabro, J. J. (1963). Vertebral wedge osteotomy correction of rheumatoid (ankylosing) spondylitis. *J. Am. Med. Assoc.*, **186,** 627–31

59. McMaster, M. J. (1985). A technique for lumbar spinal osteotomy in ankylosing spondylitis. *J. Bone Jt Surg.*, **67B,** 204–10

60. Kornberg, M. (1985). Lumbar spinal osteotomy. *Orthop. Rev.*, **14**, 59–67
61. Styblo, K., Bossers, G. Th. M. and Slot, G. H. (1985). Osteotomy for kyphosis in ankylosing spondylitis. *Acta Orthop. Scand.*, **56**, 294–7
62. Urist, M. R. (1958). Osteotomy of the cervical spine. *J. Bone Jt Surg.*, **40A**, 833–43
63. William, F., Taylor, A. R., Arden, G. P. and Edwards, D. H. (1977). Arthroplasty of the hip in ankylosing spondylitis. *J. Bone Jt Surg.*, **59B**, 393–7
64. Bisla, R. S., Ranawat, C. S. and Inglis, A. E. (1976). Total hip replacement in patients with ankylosing spondylitis with involvement of the hip. *J. Bone Jt Surg.*, **58A**, 233–8
65. Reginster, J. Y., Damas, P. and Franchimont, P. (1985). Anaesthetic risks in osteoarticular disorders. *Clin. Rheumatol.*, **4**, 30–8
66. Wittmann, F. W. (1986). Anaesthesia for hip replacement in ankylosing spondylitis. *J. R. Soc. Med.*, **79**, 457–9

# INDEX

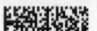